Chest Pain— Is It Your Heart?

David Andres Ph

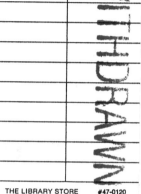

Published by Colco Publishing
P.O. Box 35099
Houston, TX 77235-5099

Printed and bound in the United States of America

Library of Congress Catalog Number 87-070554

ISBN 0-9618345-0-1

ACKNOWLEDGMENT

The author wishes to express his appreciation to Mr. Van S. Newman and to Mr. Ron Garrison for the excellent drawings and diagrams they have created and to Rhonda Love Shemtov, Janet Andres, and Nita Andres for their careful editing of the text.

Much of the information in these chapters comes from medical books, journal articles, and colleagues too numerous to list. The author gratefully acknowledges his indebtedness to all those sources.

The author wishes especially to thank the patients he has seen in over 100,000 face-to-face hands-on visits during his 35 years of medical practice. They are the most important contributors to this book and the reason it was written.

WARNING

NO ONE SHOULD ATTEMPT TO DIAGNOSE OR TREAT CHEST PAIN IN HIMSELF OR ANYONE ELSE ON THE BASIS OF ANYTHING IN THIS OR ANY OTHER BOOK. IF YOU HAVE CHEST PAIN SEE YOUR DOCTOR AS SOON AS POSSIBLE.

CONTENTS

PREFACE

This book is for the person with chest pain who wants to know what is happening to him, why, and what can be done about it. We are far from having all the answers, but our knowledge is increasing rapidly.

The book is not designed to be read straight through. A detailed table of contents is provided. It is suggested that the reader go first to any section that particularly interests him; he can consult other sections as the need arises.

Some words we use can have several different meanings; a few others are medical terms for which there are no easy substitutes. We also use some abbreviations. The glossary at the back explains these words and abbreviations in plain language.

"He," "him," and "his" mean "he or she," "him or her," and "his or hers" except where the text makes it very plain that we are referring to males only. Coronary artery disease is the number one killer of women as it is of men, although women tend to be affected at a later age.

A summary begins each chapter. The summaries are intended only to introduce the subjects covered; the subjects themselves are explained in more detail in the bodies of the chapters.

The chapters are extensively cross-referenced. Every reader will be familiar with some of the subjects we discuss, but almost no one will be well acquainted with all of them. Cross-referencing makes it easier to start anywhere and go to other sections as desired.

Medical diagnosis and treatment are not all or nothing at all propositions. They usually involve a process of zeroing in. Often the process is rapid, accurate, and highly successful; sometimes it is lengthy, time consuming, and not satisfactory.

This is not a how-to book. No one should attempt to diagnose or treat chest pain on the basis of anything he reads in this book or any other book or books. Anyone with chest pain should see a physician as soon as possible.

FACTS ABOUT HEART PAIN

Pain in the chest going to the left arm does not always mean heart trouble. This type of pain may come from a number of other sources including diaphragm, esophagus, chest and arm muscles, and emotional stress (chapters I and IV).

Gas in the stomach or intestine does not press on the heart. Even if the intestine or stomach bulges into the chest through a hiatus hernia, which is a defect in the diaphragm, no heart problems result (chapters III and IV).

Heart pain is not always severe. It may be moderate or mild. Heart pain is caused by not enough blood reaching part of the heart; episodes of insufficient blood supply to part of the heart may occur with no pain of any kind (chapters II and VII).

It is never too late to:
stop smoking
control high blood pressure
control diabetes
control blood cholesterol
control weight
start exercising
watch your diet
These are all true whether you have heart trouble or not. Many people live normal lives for many years after they develop serious heart problems. Often moderate changes in life patterns can make a big difference in health. Everyone should stop smoking; the other factors should be controlled under medical supervision (chapter IX).

Chapter One

CHEST PAIN—IS IT YOUR HEART?

A. Summary
Chest pain may come from the heart or from one or more of a number of other structures near the heart. Pain from the heart, which we will call cardiac pain, may be associated with the threat of cardiac arrest (chapter II) and sudden death. This is rarely true of other kinds of chest pain. Distinguishing between cardiac and non-cardiac chest pain is very important. Except for the possible effect of added general stress, non-cardiac pain is not connected to the heart and does not harm it in any way.

In all or almost all cases cardiac pain is caused by an insufficient supply of blood to part of the heart. There is no good evidence for any other cause of cardiac pain, but there is no way to rule out the possibility completely. Ischemia is the word we use for insufficient blood supply to any part of the body. Ischemic heart disease is usually caused by narrowing of the blood vessels supplying the heart—the coronary arteries. The cause of the narrowing in the great majority of cases is atherosclerosis, which is the deposit of cholesterol (chapter IX) and related substances in the inner layers of the walls of blood vessels.

While the fundamental problem is atherosclerosis, narrowing may be made worse at any time by one or both of 2 additional processes: spasm and blood clot formation. Spasm is the abnormal contraction of muscle cells (chapter III) in the walls of arteries; clotting is the conversion of liquid blood to the solid form.

Currently there are about 6 million people in the U.S. who have episodes of chest pain coming from their hearts. They have ischemic heart disease. About 550,000 people die every year as a result of this problem; 350,000 of the 550,000 die before they can reach a hospital. In many cases death is caused by electrical instability (chapter II, cardiac arrest) resulting from a relatively minor block in a coronary artery branch. Such blocks can often be corrected before they cause serious trouble; we will discuss methods of correction later. These are truly "hearts too good to die."

Many more than 6 million people have episodes of non-cardiac chest pain every year. The cause of the pain is often obvious; many times, however, it is mistaken for cardiac pain.

We will look at 5 case studies to illustrate some of the kinds of chest pain we see. In 3 of these patients the pain was cardiac; in the other 2 it was not. The steps in the diagnosis and treatment of these patients will be discussed in more detail throughout the book.

The single most important means we have for evaluating chest pain is the medical history—what the patient tells us about the pain. We use many tests and procedures, but the medical history, when it can be obtained, is the backbone of our decision-making process.

Neither the history nor any test we use will distinguish cardiac from non-cardiac pain every time. We have no perfect tests. Since we cannot get a perfect answer by combining imperfect tests (chapter V), we use expressions like "almost always" and "almost never" but almost never say "always" or "never."

B. Introduction

All parts of the body need blood to live and work properly; the heart is no exception. Although other mechanisms cannot be ruled out completely, at least in nearly all cases cardiac pain is caused by insufficient blood supply to part of the heart. This may seem strange, since normally all the blood in the body makes a trip through the heart about once every minute. Unfortunately, the heart has no way of getting at the blood passing through its chambers. The blood it needs must come by way of its own small vessels. The vessels supplying the heart are called coronary arteries (chapter III). The decreased blood supply causing pain usually results from narrowing or blockage of one or more of these arteries or their branches.

Coronary artery narrowing takes place by one or more of 3 related processes: 1) atherosclerosis 2) spasm 3) blood clot formation (chapter II). Atherosclerosis is the fundamental problem; it is the collection of cholesterol and related chemical compounds in the inner layers of the walls of the arteries. These collections form mounds or plaques which narrow the arterial channels. Spasm and/or clot formation usually happen in arteries with preexisting atherosclerosis. They further narrow or completely close the affected artery.

Non-cardiac chest pain can come from a number of organs and tissues in and around the chest. Furthermore, each of these structures may become painful from a variety of causes. Distinguishing cardiac from non-cardiac pain is extremely important. Not only do we have to know the origin of the pain to treat it properly, but cardiac pain is in general much more dangerous and much more likely to demand immediate attention than the non-cardiac variety. Non-cardiac chest pain may or may not be caused by serious disease. However, with the few exceptions we will discuss in chapter II, it is very rarely associated with the threat of sudden death.

Five case studies are presented to tie our discussions to real people. We will give the steps in presentation, diagnosis, and treatment as they actually happened. Throughout the book we will be referring to these steps with more detailed explanations of what was done and why.

We will try to avoid unfamiliar language where possible. However, more and more medical terms are coming into general use as people increasingly take an active part in the managment of their own illnesses. Many terms are explained in the text as they appear; a glossary is also included for quick reference.

Two words have already been introduced. The first, "ischemia," means insufficient blood supply. "Ischemic heart disease" is heart disease caused by insufficient blood supply

13

to part of that organ. Ischemic heart disease is the central subject of this book. The second word, "spasm," has a number of possible meanings. We will use it in a restricted medical sense to mean inappropriate muscle cell contraction. A common example is a leg cramp. The cells in a leg muscle contract but do not relax normally. This is felt as prolonged painful tightening of the muscle. The walls of arteries also contain muscle cells, although of a different kind than leg muscle; they are wrapped around the artery. These cells normally regulate the size of the arteries, helping to distribute blood properly to the body. In some cases these cells go into spasm; they contract too much for too long. This constricts the artery, causing ischemia—insufficient blood supply to the part of the body the artery supplies. Coronary artery spasm is one cause of cardiac ischemia.

C. Cardiac pain, atherosclerosis, and cardiac arrest

1. The problem

This year about 6 million people in the U.S. will have one or more episodes of chest pain originating in their hearts. About 550,000 of these people will die this year, over half of them in one hour or less of the onset of their pain or collapse. In the great majority of instances, coronary artery atherosclerosis is the basic cause of the pain and cardiac arrest (chapter II).

2. Coronary atherosclerosis, chest pain, and consequences

Coronary arteries are the vessels that supply the heart with blood (chapter III). Atherosclerosis in these arteries usually appears as localized heaped-up mounds we call plaques. The plaques cause a spotty narrowing of the arterial channels; this narrowing decreases the flow of blood to the heart. Too little blood to the heart causes pain.

Decreased blood supply to the heart may also cause electrical changes leading to abnormal patterns of heartbeat, up to and including cardiac arrest. Cardiac arrest is the sudden and complete stoppage of effective heartbeats. If the heart stops beating, no body organs receive blood. Death results in a very few minutes unless adequate heart action can be restored.

3. Ischemic heart disease

When blood supply to the heart drops enough to cause pain, electrical disturbances, or cardiac arrest, the patient is said to have "ischemic heart disease" or "cardiac ischemia" or "coronary heart disease." Practically speaking, these terms are used interchangeably. They all describe the situation of inadequate blood flow to parts of the heart. Ischemic heart disease may result from coronary atherosclerosis alone or atherosclerosis plus coronary spasm and/or blood clot formation (thrombosis).

Atherosclerosis is probably reversible to some extent, at least in its earlier stages. There is evidence that the plaques do get smaller at times. Spasm and clot formation are definitely reversible. Spasm can very often be controlled with medication. Clot formation can be slowed and in some cases clots can be dissolved. We will discuss treatment and prevention much more in chapters VIII and IX.

4. "Hearts too good to die"

Ischemic heart disease is our number one killer. It accounts for more deaths than all forms of cancer combined. It kills over 10 times as many people each year as auto accidents. Its overall price tag in the U.S. is about 60 billion dollars yearly.

Usually, chest pain and/or cardiac arrest are the only evidence the patient has of the problem. Many people who have cardiac arrests do not have widespread disease of their hearts or coronary arteries. Their atherosclerosis is well localized and is or would have been treatable in one of several ways. Dr. Claude Beck, a pioneer American heart surgeon, invented the phrase that sums it up—"hearts too good to die."

C. Non-cardiac chest pain

This year many more than 6 million people in the U.S. will have episodes of chest pain not originating in their hearts. Most of these will be recognized as "gas" or "indigestion" and more or less ignored.

Sometimes non-cardiac chest pain is due to disease; the disease may be minor or serious. Regardless of its cause or severity, non-cardiac chest pain differs from cardiac chest pain in one extremely important respect. Except for problems originating in the large blood vessels around the heart (aorta, pulmonary artery, and great veins), non-cardiac chest pain is very rarely associated with the threat of sudden death. Deciding which kind of pain is present is vital.

D. Examples: patients with chest pain
We are going to give the case histories of 5 patients. The first 3 illustrate the major ways cardiac pain presents: angina pectoris, myocardial infarction, and cardiac arrest. The others represent 2 of the many different forms of non-cardiac chest pain. The cases were chosen because they are reasonably typical and allow us to discuss a wide range of diagnostic and therapeutic procedures. The first 2 have happy endings, but this must not be taken to mean that all patients treated like this will do as well. Treatment must be individualized for each patient and, unfortunately, happy endings can never be assured.

Our emphasis is on patient history. The single most important factor in deciding where the pain is coming from is what the patient tells the doctor. We almost always do additional tests, but our immediate decisions about treatment are based on what we hear from the patient and the people who bring him in. This of course does not apply to the patient who is unconscious or otherwise unable to talk coherently. In those situations we operate under a different set of rules.

1. Angina pectoris
The distinguishing characteristic of angina pectoris is the lack of permanent gross heart damage from the episodes of ischemia. Pain and electrocardiographic evidence of ischemia are present, but these disappear when the situation causing the ischemia is relieved. Whether episodes of angina can cause microscopic areas of scar formation is a subject of debate.

Patient #1
A 50 year old man began to notice pain in his chest and left arm during moderately severe physical exertion such as moving boxes and equipment around at work. He described the pain as an ache or pressure; sometimes it had a burning quality. It did not come on with the first motion, but only after a variable period of effort. It was not sharp and was not severe. However, it did make him stop any activity until it went away, usually in about 2 to 4 minutes. The pain was not

made worse by deep breathing, coughing, or any change in position. It was not affected in any way by specific movements of his arms or body. His chest was not tender. His physical examination was completely normal.

This patient's history was sufficient to establish the diagnosis of angina pectoris. He was started on treatment immediately. He later had a resting electrocardiogram (chapter VII) which was normal. This was followed by a stress test (chapter VII) which was inconclusive. As is often the case in ischemic heart disease, these tests were initially not helpful. He was given a prescription for nitroglycerin (chapter VIII) to put under his tongue. Later he was given longer acting nitro compounds to take regularly. These worked for a while. However, his exercise and stress tolerance decreased gradually over the next 13 years in spite of additional medications and treatment. At 13 years from the time he first had pain he could walk only one block before chest discomfort caused him to stop.

This patient had classical stable angina pectoris (chapter II). The buildup of cholesterol and related compounds in his coronary arteries was proceeding at a very slow rate. At first his heart was getting enough blood to sustain a fairly heavy work load. As time went on, more cholesterol and related materials were deposited in the arterial walls. Eventually the maximum amount of blood the narrowed channels could deliver to the affected part of his heart was little more than enough to maintain a resting level of activity. The medicines he took helped at first by decreasing the load on his heart and probably by dilating some of the less affected coronary arteries. With increased arterial narrowing, the medicines became less and less effective.

The patient requested that he be evaluated for bypass surgery; at that time (1975) balloon dilatation (chapter VIII) had not been developed. Coronary angiography (chapter VII) was performed; his atherosclerosis was found to be sufficiently localized so that there was a very good chance that he would benefit from bypass surgery.

Accordingly, the procedure was performed. The patient felt much better before he left the hospital. Within 2 months after surgery he was able to walk a mile in 15 minutes. Currently (11 years after surgery, at age 74) he walks 2 miles daily without any symptoms of angina. He still has pain at the site of his incision (the middle of his breastbone) at times.

This was an excellent result. Not all patients who have the operation do as well. We will discuss the procedure and results in more detail in chapter VIII.

2. Myocardial infarction

Myocardium is heart muscle; infarction is death of tissue because of insufficient blood supply. Myocardial infarction therefore means death of heart muscle because of insufficient blood supply. The dead muscle is eventually replaced by scar tissue.

Patient #2

A 54 year old man had the sudden (over to 2 to 3 minutes) onset of severe pain in the middle of his chest while driving to work. A similar episode about a month before had gone away by itself in about 30 minutes. This time the pain was much worse and gave no indication that it was going to stop.

The patient drove straight to the hospital. On arrival he described his pain as crushing and pressure-like. It did not go to either arm or any other part of his body. It did not change with motion, change of position, or deep breathing. His chest wall was not tender.

The pattern of this patient's illness was a common one for acute myocardial infarction. In most cases this condition is caused by coronary artery thrombosis; that is, a blood clot forms on a preexisting atherosclerotic plaque in a coronary artery. Treatment was started immediately, based on the patient's description of his pain. An electrocardiogram was obtained; it showed changes typical of acute myocardial infarction (chapter VII). Sometimes the electrocardiogram is normal in this situation. Our patient would have been treated for a myocardial infarction no matter what his electrocardiogram looked like.

As soon as the patient's history, blood pressure, and heart rate were obtained he was given nitroglycerin under his tongue. The nitroglycerin was repeated in 2 minutes. The medication had no effect on his pain. While he was being given the medicine, oxygen and an intravenous infusion were being started. He was given morphine for pain and lidocaine and a beta blocking agent to stabilize his heart action (chapter VIII).

It was explained to the patient that he appeared to be

developing a myocardial infarction and that there was available on an experimental basis a clot dissolving agent (streptokinase, chapter VIII) which had been showing great promise in cases like his. The risks, mainly allergy and delayed bleeding, were explained to him. He was asked about recent surgery, bleeding problems, and other things which might make the use of the medication inadvisable. The patient requested that the medication be given. Accordingly, an intravenous infusion of streptokinase was started (chapter VIII).

As we said, the initial electrocardiogram showed the characteristic changes of a type of myocardial infarction. Part of this pattern, a change indicating cardiac ischemia, was being duplicated on the cardiac monitor attached to the patient (chapter VII). About 20 minutes after the streptokinase was started the patient had a small flurry of rapid heartbeats. The ischemic pattern on the monitor disappeared and was replaced by a normal one. At the same time, the patient's pain disappeared; he said he felt fine.

He was kept on medication and was watched carefully for the next 2 days. He had no pain and felt well during this time. Cardiography and coronary angiography (chapter VII) were then performed. The heart walls and heart motion appeared normal. A single atherosclerotic area suitable for balloon dilatation (PTCA, chapter VIII) was seen. The constriction was dilated without problems; 2 days later the patient went home. He was back at full activity and work 10 days after his attack. Currently (21 months after his attack) he is completely free of symptoms; his only medicine is a beta blocker (chapter VIII).

This also was a very good result. Clot dissolution is still very new and is considered largely experimental. This patient was an excellent candidate. Streptokinase was started in less than one hour from the onset of his pain. Currently we can expect 50 to 60% good results if treatment is started within about 4 hours of the onset of symptoms. These figures will hopefully improve as better clot dissolving agents are released. Although the clot itself can be dissolved much later, it is becoming evident that residual heart damage may increase with time, even within the 4 hour period.

With early treatment good results can be obtained in patients with extensive coronary atherosclerosis. Angiograms are now frequently done the day after streptokinase treatment, with balloon dilatation or bypass surgery the following day. It should be borne in mind that even if the clot is dissolved, streptokinase does nothing for the atherosclerosis that started the clot. Treatment and timing must always be individualized for each patient by a competent doctor. However, if further procedures are indicated, there appears to be good reason to do them as soon as the patient's condition makes them advisable.

3. Cardiac arrest
This is the most disastrous complication of ischemic heart disease. The heart stops suddenly and the patient dies unless heart action is restored in a very few minutes. Often this is an electrical problem (chapter II); there may be little residual permanent damage to the heart muscle if the patient is resuscitated. However, cardiac arrest tends to recur; the recurrence rate can be decreased with proper treatment (chapter VIII).

Patient #3
A 62 year old man was brought to the hospital emergency department by fire department paramedics with cardiopulmonary resuscitation (CPR; rhythmic chest compression to pump blood and rhythmic inflation of the lungs in order to supply oxygen) in progress. He had been playing golf and had just started his cart for the next hole when he slumped over the wheel. When they arrived at the golf course the paramedics found no audible heartbeat and no breathing. In spite of medications and electric shocks his heart could not be restarted. Before playing golf that morning he had casually told one of his golfing partners that he had been having chest pain off and on for 3 days. He had not seen a doctor or mentioned the problem to anyone else.

About 350,000 of the 550,000 people who die yearly in the U.S. of ischemic heart disease will have a history something like this; 75 to 85% of them will have had chest pain at some time prior to their cardiac arrests. The arrest itself frequently occurs suddenly without warning; at other times there is chest pain of variable duration. As we said, many of these people do not have widespread disease; their hearts can be restarted and function well if we can get them soon enough. With the present state of our knowledge and practice, the number of successful resuscitations drops rapidly if basic life support is not started in 4 minutes and advanced life support in 8 minutes from the time of arrest. Research is currently being done on ways to extend these times.

Basic life support consists of mouth to mouth breathing to get air into the patient's lungs and regular chest compressions to pump blood to the heart, brain, and rest of the body. The American Heart Association sponsors basic life support courses throughout the country. Ideally, everyone from the age of 9 up should take such a course. Basic life support is a fundamental key to saving the lives of some of the 350,000 people who die like patient #3 every year.

Advanced cardiac life support involves the use of drugs, electric shock, and special procedures to assist breathing. It requires equipment ordinarily not available outside hospitals and ambulances, as well as extensive training of personnel. A major problem is to get this type of assistance to the patient soon enough.

4. Non-cardiac pain; the musculoskeletal system

Patient #4

A 39 year old man came to the hospital emergency department complaining of left chest and left arm pain of 4 or 5 hours' duration. He said that the pain was made worse by raising his arm or moving his shoulder, but not by deep breathing or coughing. There was tenderness of the left chest and left shoulder muscles. The tip of his left shoulder was especially sensitive. The patient at first denied any unusual lifting, straining, or other physical activity. On persistent questioning he remembered a long and strenuous tennis session 2 days previously.

In spite of repeated reassurances the patient remained very much concerned that his heart was causing the pain. An electrocardiogram was obtained; it was normal.

This patient had inflammation of a shoulder tendon plus strain of his shoulder and chest muscles. As many people who engage in strenuous sports know, it may take as long as 3 days for pain to show up after unaccustomed heavy physical exertion. Pain aggravated by specific movements of the arm or chest comes from the muscles of the chest wall, arm, or shoulder: it does not come from the heart and is not a sign of ischemic heart disease. This type of pain must be carefully differentiated from pain brought on by a period of exertion which increases the load on the heart. Both types of pain may

21

occur in the same person. Careful questioning and examination usually make it evident that there are 2 different types of pain brought on in entirely different ways.

5. Chest wall pain; "periapical fatigue," "neurocirculatory asthenia"

Patient #5

A 25 year old man came to the emergency department complaining of chest pain and fluttering of his heart. The pain was sharp and localized to his left chest; occasionally it went down his left arm. The pain was not made worse by coughing, deep breathing, or changes in position. His left chest wall was tender. He had been having episodes of pain like this for 3 or 4 years; they usually lasted for several hours and disappeared by themselves. They were not brought on by physical exertion. He had been having emotional problems for years but could not relate the pain directly to periods of increased emotional stress.

The patient had seen other doctors who had done electrocardiograms and other tests. They told him that he did have heartbeat irregularities but no heart disease of any kind. (Cardiac rhythm disturbances sometimes mean heart disease and sometimes do not. Almost everyone has an occasional extra beat: some people with normal hearts have many.) This patient's electrocardiogram confirmed the presence of extra heartbeats which did not indicate heart disease (chapter VII).

The 2 names given above for this condition translate into "tiredness around the tip of the heart" and "nerve-muscle weakness." Both terms are meaningless, as are all other names attached to this problem. The mechanism for the production of the pain is not known. The pain has a very strong emotional basis. Nevertheless, it is real. It is in the patient's chest, not his head. The pain is not cardiac; it is not associated with any threat to life or physical well-being. Treatment depends mainly on the nature and extent of the patient's emotional problems.

There are many additional kinds of non-cardiac chest pain (chapter IV). Usually the history and physical examination are enough to allow us to pinpoint the source of the discomfort. Sometimes, however, non-cardiac pain may resemble cardiac pain so closely that only admission to the hospital, observation, and adequate testing (chapter VII) enable us to tell the difference.

E. Problems with the history

The patient's history is our single most important diagnostic tool. This has good and bad points. On the plus side, we can start treatment immediately; all we need is a patient able to talk and tell us what is wrong. On the minus side, people vary tremendously. Some have higher physical or psychological pain thresholds than others. Even in people who seem to have about the same pain tolerance there are great differences in pain caused by the same heart damage. The reason for these differences is not known. As we will see later, painless episodes of cardiac ischemia occur (chapter VII).

People also differ in their ability and willingness to describe their symptoms. Some paint detailed and accurate word pictures; others communicate mainly with grunts. Finally, pain coming from other chest or abdominal organs may mimic that coming from the heart.

For these reasons the history, useful as it is, is far from perfect as a means of distinguishing cardiac from non-cardiac pain. We almost always use additional tests; these are not perfect either. We cannot get perfect answers by combining imperfect tests, although we can decrease our margin of error by increasing the number of such tests (chapter V). We cannot say "never" or "always."

Chapter Two

CARDIAC PAIN, CORONARY ATHEROSCLEROSIS, AND SUDDEN DEATH

A. Summary

Most if not all cardiac pain is caused by inadequate blood supply to the heart. We call this ischemic heart disease. The most common cause is atherosclerotic narrowing of the blood vessels supplying the heart. Characteristics of the pain that help us decide whether it is cardiac or not are type of pain, location, severity, duration, and things that make it better or worse. Of these the type of pain and things that make it better or worse are the most important. Duration and time sequence sometimes help. Location and severity can be misleading.

The deposition of cholesterol and related materials in artery walls is almost always gradual; it frequently progresses through adult life. Pain usually does not appear until the diameter of a blood vessel is decreased at least 50%. Ischemic heart disease is a late complication of this slow process.

Ischemic heart disease appears in one or more of 3 forms: angina pectoris, myocardial infarction, or cardiac arrest.

The ischemia of angina pectoris is reversible; it comes and goes. It results from a mismatch between the amount of blood the heart needs and the amount of blood it gets. In the presence of coronary artery disease the mismatch may be caused by an increase load on the heart from such things as exercise, emotional stress, or eating. The heart has to work harder and needs more blood. The narrowed coronary arteries cannot carry an adequate amount. When the stress causing the increased heart load stops, heart work decreases, the blood supply again becomes adequate, and the pain stops. The arterial narrowing is usually produced by atherosclerosis with the possible addition of arterial spasm or a temporary clot.

Myocardial infarction means death of heart muscle with eventual replacement by scar tissue. The most common cause is a blood clot forming in an atherosclerotic segment of artery, blocking the artery completely. In this case the body does not dissolve the clot. If the clot is not dissolved in a short time (in a few hours at most) by one of the medicines that have recently become available, decreased blood supply causes permanent heart damage. The pain of myocardial infarction is like that of angina pectoris, but is usually more intense. It does not go away by itself and is not relieved by medicines that work for angina.

Cardiac arrest is the sudden stoppage of effective heartbeat. No blood is pumped to any part of the body, including the brain and heart itself. The patient dies unless effective heartbeat is restored within a few minutes. This grace period can be made longer, sometimes up to an hour or two, if adequate cardiopulmonary resuscitation is started immediately. Arrest sometimes occurs because so much heart muscle has been damaged that there is not enough left for effective contraction. More commonly, the problem is electrical. Damaged tissue sends out irregular electrical impulses which cause the heart to quiver (ventricular fibrillation) rather than contract effectively. If normal electrical activity can be restarted soon enough (by electric shock) the residual damage may be slight.

The other common causes of chest pain which may be associated with sudden death are aortic aneurysm, dissecting aortic aneurysm, pulmonary embolism, and tension pneumothorax. These all directly or indirectly involve the large blood vessels carrying blood to and from the heart.

The aorta is the single large blood vessel leaving the left side of the heart to carry blood to the entire body. An aneurysm is a blister-like weakened area in the wall of a blood vessel. Aortic aneurysms are usually caused by atherosclerosis. If the blister expands suddenly or tears, severe pain results. A tear may also result in massive blood loss and sudden death.

The problem in dissecting aneurysm is slightly different. A break in the lining of the aorta allows blood to seep in between the layers of the aortic wall. The separation of layers causes severe pain. The outer wall may also tear, resulting in massive blood loss.

The pulmonary artery is the vessel carrying blood from the right heart to the lungs. Sometimes a blood clot breaks loose from the veins in the leg or groin and lodges in the main pulmonary artery or one of its branches. All the blood in the body passes through the main pulmonary artery on its way to the lungs, so a large clot may shut down all circulation (chapter III).

Pneumothorax is a condition in which air escapes from a tear in the lung and collects in the chest cavity. Most of the time this causes only pain and some shortness of breath. If air continues to build up it may push the heart and large blood vessels out of the midline and interfere seriously with the flow of blood. This is a tension pneumothorax. Since it is usually associated with chest trauma and has distinctive physical signs, it is rarely mistaken for ischemic heart disease.

In general, each of these 4 conditions causes sufficiently severe symptoms that the patient is unlikely to delay getting medical attention. With the possible exception of some cases of pulmonary embolism they do not usually present serious diagnostic problems.

B. Cardiac pain

Most if not all cardiac pain is caused by an inadequate blood supply to part of the heart. This condition, ischemic heart disease, is usually caused by atherosclerotic narrowing, spasm, and/or clots in one or more segments of the coronary arterial tree. The most important factor in deciding whether the pain is cardiac is how the patient describes it. Characteristics that need to be considered are what kind of pain is it, where is it, how bad is it, what makes it better or worse, and how long does it last.

1. Character

This is extremely important. Cardiac pain is rarely described as sharp, needle like, piercing, stabbing, or knife like. The most common descriptive terms are aching, dull, crushing, or pressure like. The patient may say he does not feel pain, just an uncomfortable squeeze or pressure. Sometimes the sensation is described as a deep burn. Commonly but not always the patient stops all physical activity even if the pain is mild.

2. Intensity

This is of very little help. Both cardiac and non-cardiac pain can be anything from very mild to very severe. Intensity of the pain has very little to do with the severity of the underlying illness. Esophageal spasm caused by a temporary irritation can cause severe chest pain; a large myocardial infarction may cause only mild discomfort. Some episodes of cardiac ischemia produce no symptoms at all. The patient does not know that he is having trouble and only electrocardiographic changes show that there is or has been a problem. However, the patient who has painless episodes of ischemia usually has others that show characteristic pain patterns (chapter VII).

3. Location

Although most cardiac pain occurs in the middle of the chest in front, so does much non-cardiac pain. Location is frequently not helpful. Cardiac and non-cardiac pain may show up in the front or the back of the chest as well as the arm, neck, or jaw on either the right or the left side. Occasionally cardiac pain is felt in the upper abdomen below the ribs. Pain in the left chest going to the left arm may or may not have anything to do with the heart. Patients #4 and #5 (chapter I) had 2 different kinds of non-cardiac chest pain; both had pain in the left chest and left arm.

4. Aggravation and alleviation

What brings the pain on, what gets rid of it, what makes it better, and what makes it worse are factors of primary importance. If nothing changes it, that too is important. In classic angina pectoris, pain is brought on by physical exertion, heavy eating, emotional stress, cold weather, or some combination of these. Each factor increases the body's requirement for energy and therefore for oxygen. The heart must supply the blood which carries the oxygen, so it must work harder. When the heart in turn requires more oxygen than can be supplied by the amount of blood getting through the narrowed coronary arteries, pain results. Usually the patient stops what he is doing (if he can), the load on the heart decreases, and the heart's requirement for blood decreases. As cardiac demand drops enough so that it can be met by coronary blood flow, the pain stops. This pattern of pain created by increased work load, then relieved by rest, is so characteristic that it establishes the diagnosis of ischemic heart disease. Some forms of angina, however, do not show this pain pattern. They will be discussed later in this chapter as variant angina and unstable angina.

The patient's history must be taken carefully to make sure that the pain is not due to some specific or repeated motion of the arm or some part of the body; pain brought on by such specific movements is due to muscle, joint, or related problems (patient #4, chapter I).

Nitroglycerin and some other medications frequently relieve anginal pain by decreasing the load on the heart and possibly by dilating coronary arteries. Since these medications may also relieve pain from the esophagus, we have to be careful in interpreting their effects. Patients who develop myocardial infarcts (death of heart tissue from ischemia) rarely have pain relief from nitroglycerin or similar medications.

5. Duration
Each form of ischemic heart disease has a more or less specific pattern as far as duration is concerned. The pain of classical angina pectoris comes on in 2 or 3 minutes when a high enough stress level is reached; it rarely lasts more than 5 or 10 minutes after the stress is removed. It usually disappears even more rapidly in response to nitroglycerin. The pain of unstable angina may last 30 minutes or more; it may come on and leave for no apparent reason. The pain of myocardial infarction lasts days if untreated and often even with treatment.

C. Atherosclerosis and its complications

1. The atherosclerotic process
Atherosclerosis is the deposit of cholesterol and related materials under the inside linings of the walls of arteries. These deposits usually build up in localized spots called plaques. The plaques are almost always on one side of the artery; the other side may be relatively normal until late. The

deposition of these materials is usually gradual; in most cases it seems to go on for the adult life of the individual. The .arterial segment narrows until blood flow is seriously restricted and the patient begins to have the symptoms of ischemic heart disease. Chapters VIII and IX will go into more detail on the causes, treatment, and prevention of atherosclerosis.

Symptoms do not usually appear until the inside diameter of the artery is decreased by 50% or more. There are 2 reasons for this. First, the coronary circulation has a lot of reserve capacity; it has to have to handle loads induced by extreme exertion or stress. Secondly, at a certain degree of narrowing, small changes in diameter cause large changes in flow. For those interested in numbers, flow at constant pressure varies as the fourth power of the diameter. Generally, all forms of ischemic heart disease are late complications of a process that has been going on for a long time.

2. Ischemic heart disease: angina pectoris, myocardial infarction, cardiac arrest

2.a. Angina pectoris

The distinguishing feature of angina is that the ischemia is reversible. No patches of heart damage large enough to be seen by the unaided eye result from the attacks, although there is some question that irreversible microscopic damage may occur.

2.a.1. Classical angina

In classical angina pectoris, chest pain comes on with stress such as physical exertion, cold, heavy eating, or emotional tension. Stress increases cardiac work load. Inadequate blood supply to the heart for the work it must perform causes pain. Atherosclerotic narrowing of parts of the coronary tree is the usual but not the only possible cause.

At first the pain comes on only with relatively severe stress, physical or emotional. Over the years the plaques build up, restricting flow more and more. Correspondingly less stress is required for cardiac demand to exceed the limited supply of blood. The pain is still usually relieved by rest and/or medicines such as nitroglycerin. Patient #1 (chapter I) is a typical example of someone with stable classical angina. "Stable" refers to the fact that his illness was slowly progressive over many years with no sudden changes; "classical" means that it demonstrated the most common pattern, pain aggravated by increased cardiac load and relieved by rest.

2.a.2. Variant angina

Sometimes angina does not fit the classical picture. The walls of arteries are circled by muscle cells. Abnormal contraction of these cells causes arteries to constrict inappropriately, a condition we call spasm. Spasm usually relaxes before it can cause permanent damage. However, in some cases it appears to be the precipitating event for cardiac arrest and possibly for myocardial infarction. While it is present, spasm limits blood flow to parts of the heart just as does atherosclerotic narrowing. Spasm usually occurs in coronary artery systems with well defined atherosclerosis. It is frequently not related to any exertion. No one knows why it shows up when it does. It may occur at rest or during sleep. Variant angina is also sometimes called Prinzmetal's angina, although there is some argument about terminology. Spastic arteries relax and dilate in response to nitroglycerin and related medications as well as to drugs called calcium channel blockers (chapter VIII), so these are effective treatments for variant angina.

Probably related to spasm is the occurrence of "walk-through angina." In this situation the patient starts an activity and develops anginal pain. If he rests for a few minutes and restarts the activity at the same exertion level, the pain does not come back no matter how long he continues. In other cases he may not even need to rest; the pain may disappear and not return even if he continues the activity without interruption.

The usual progress of angina may be interrupted at any time by the development of unstable angina, myocardial infarction, or cardiac arrest.

2.a.3. Unstable angina.

At times angina does not follow the classic pattern of gradually getting worse. Progress of the disease seems to accelerate, so that the patient deteriorates over weeks or even days. This condition is called unstable angina or preinfarctional angina or coronary insufficiency, all names for the same process.

Doctors have very recently been able to look inside the

31

coronary arteries of living patients with fiberoptic instruments. These are long flexible bundles of thin glass rods which carry light from their tips to the observer's eye. In classical angina the predictable bulge of the atherosclerotic plaque is seen. Patients with unstable angina also have plaques, but on these blood clots are seen forming and breaking up in an irregular manner, causing variable amounts of obstruction.

Ischemia at this stage is still reversible; no permanent damage to the heart is observed. However, as implied by the name, the condition is unstable. The chance of progression to a myocardial infarction is great.

2.b. Myocardial infarction

Myocardial infarction means heart muscle (myocardium) death due to decreased blood supply (infarction). Tissues of the heart other than muscle are also usually involved, so the term is not a complete label. In most cases the condition is caused by the formation of a blood clot on an atherosclerotic plaque. Unlike the clots of unstable angina, this one does not break up. It usually stops up the artery completely. Unless the clot is dissolved within a very few hours by one of the medicines that have recently become available (chapter VIII), the sudden drop in blood supply results in permanent damage to the heart. A part of the heart muscle dies and is eventually replaced by scar tissue.

The pain of myocardial infarction has the same character as that described for angina but is usually more severe. Sometimes, however, it is mild and occasionally it is completely absent. When present the pain is not relieved by nitroglycerin or similar medicines; usually strong narcotics are required. Without treatment the pain usually lasts for days.

2.c. Cardiac arrest

The most dreaded complication of ischemic heart disease is cardiac arrest. The heart stops beating, no blood flows to the brain and body, and death results in a very few minutes unless the heartbeat is restarted.

Not long ago the process was considered straightforward. A blood clot formed in a coronary artery, not enough blood got to the heart, and the heart stopped beating from overall lack of oxygen and nutrients. This is the mechanism in some but not in most cases.

Normal heart action starts with an electrical impulse from the SA node in the right atrium (chapter III). The impulse progresses through both atria and ventricles in an orderly manner, causing an efficient coordinated contraction. However, beats can originate from parts of the heart other than the SA node. Every part of the heart is capable of initiating an impulse leading to a contraction. Heart muscle damaged but not killed by oxygen lack is especially irritable in this regard. Sometimes such muscle initiates multiple rapid irregular impulses. These spread through the heart causing irregular contractions of small muscle bundles rather than a coordinated beat. The ventricles (chapter III) start to quiver like a bag of worms rather than beating normally; in this state the heart pumps no blood. This is called ventricular fibrillation. As we said, it is fatal in a few minutes unless it is stopped (usually by an appropriate electric shock) and coordinated heartbeats restored.

Ventricular fibrillation must be carefully distinguished from atrial fibrillation, in which only the atria (chapter III) stop their beating and quiver. Atrial fibrillation may be the result of various kinds of heart problems. It can even occur as a temporary disturbance in people with normal hearts. While it causes cardiac irregularity, it is often compatible with a full active life span even when heart disease is present.

Ventricular fibrillation is the most common disturbance causing cardiac arrest and sudden death. Although it occurs sometimes in patients with congenital or developmental heart abnormalities, coronary atherosclerosis is far and away the most common underlying problem. A large amount of damaged tissue is not necessarily present. To repeat, these often are "hearts too good to die." We will discuss what is being done about the problem in chapters VIII and IX.

Sometimes instead of fibrillating the ventricular muscle stops contracting completely. This is called asystole and is usually more difficult to reverse than ventricular fibrillation. The result is the same; no blood is pumped and death follows unless effective heartbeats can be restarted. At other times the irritable damaged tissue sends out rapid single impulses or initiates a kind of round and round circus movement of impulses. This results in the rapid inefficient beat pattern called ventricular tachycardia. Tachycardia just means rapid heartbeat. There are other forms of tachycardia which are not dangerous and may not indicate heart disease at all. This is sometimes true even of ventricular tachycardia. However, when this dysrhythmia is present in the setting of ischemic heart disease, the ventricles may or may not pump enough blood to sustain consciousness or even life. Taken together, ventricular fibrillation, asystole, and ventricular tachycardia are the immediate causes of sudden death in the great majority of cases. About 85% of cardiac sudden deaths occur in patients with known ischemic heart disease. There is no history of heart pain in the remaining 15%. See however patient #3, chapter I; not all people with chest pain tell about it.

D. Other causes of chest pain associated with sudden death

1. Ruptured aortic aneurysm
   An aneurysm is a bulging weak spot in the wall of an artery or the heart. Although they occur in other arteries, the ones we are concerned with are in the aorta (chapter III). The most common cause is, again, atherosclerosis. In the lower aorta near the legs, atherosclerosis may cause narrowing and clot formation as it does in the coronary arteries. Higher in the abdomen and in the chest the process weakens the artery and allows it to bulge. As long as it progresses slowly, the patient may be totally unaware of the presence of the aneurysm. Rapid stretching of the bulge or a blood leak causes pain. If the wall tears, a clot may seal it temporarily, there may be continuous leakage of blood into the chest, or there may be a sudden massive fatal blood loss. An expanding or leaking aneurysm is a life threatening emergency and is treated as such.
   The pain is almost always very severe. It may be felt in the chest, back, or abdomen; at times it is much like the pain of myocardial infarction. Sometimes evidence of an aneurysm can be seen on chest or abdominal x-rays or felt in the abdomen. Angiograms, which are x-rays made with materials injected into the blood vessels to outline them (chapter VII), are usually necessary to be sure of the exact nature and extent of the problem.
   The treatment for this type of aneurysm is generally surgical. It usually involves removal of the affected segment of aorta and replacement with a woven dacron tube. Other special surgical procedures may be necessary.

34

2. Dissecting aortic aneurysm

The aneurysms described above occur when all 3 layers of the wall of the aorta weaken and bulge. In a dissecting aneurysm the inner wall of the aorta cracks, allowing blood to get between the layers of the vessel and separate them. A dissecting aneurysm may rupture, with consequences such as those described in the previous section. The dissection at other times may partly or completely close off branches of the aorta, causing pain or loss of function in the organs they supply.

The pain is frequently described as tearing, in keeping with the process itself. It may be in the chest and/or up and down the back, depending on the location of the dissection. Sometimes the pain is greatly relieved by medication decreasing the patient's blood pressure and thus the stress on the arterial wall.

Treatment of this condition must be individualized. For some patients, removal of the damaged artery and replacement with a graft is best; others do better with careful control of blood pressure.

3. Pulmonary embolism

An embolus is a clot that has broken loose from its site of formation and lodged in a blood vessel some distance away. The most common sites of clot formation are the veins of the thigh and lower body; sometimes clots form in the heart itself.

A pulmonary embolus is a clot that has become lodged in the main pulmonary artery or one of its branches. A clot that completely blocks the main pulmonary artery is incompatible with life; no blood can get to the lungs or body. At the other end of the scale a small clot may lodge in a minor arterial branch and cause no symptoms. Frequently a small embolus causes a temporary episode of shortness of breath and nothing more. Damaged tissue at the outer border of the lung can cause pain when it rubs against the inner chest wall with each breath. The pain is called pleuritic (from pleura, the outer covering of the lung and the inner covering of the chest wall). The pain is sharp, made worse by breathing, and unlikely to be confused with cardiac pain.

If a larger clot stops in a major pulmonary artery branch it may cause increased pressure in the pulmonary artery system. This pressure increase may cause pain which is dull, oppressive, and much like the pain of myocardial infarction. The pain is usually accompanied by shortness of breath, which is uncommon in all but the most severe cases of myocardial infarction. Electrocardiographic changes, if they are present, are likely to be characteristic of pulmonary embolism and not myocardial infarction (chapter VII). Special x-ray and radionuclide studies (chapter VII) may demonstrate blocks in the pulmonary artery tree.

4. Tension pneumothorax
    A pneumothorax occurs when air gets between the lung and chest wall, allowing the lung to collapse to a greater or lesser extent (see chapter III on the mechanism of lung expansion). The usual source of the air is a tear in the lung. The tear may result from the rupture of a thin blister on the lung for no apparent reason (spontaneous pneumothorax). Pneumothorax may also be caused by injury. The cause of the injury may be penetrating, like a knife or a broken rib, or it may be a blow to the chest with no penetration. Physical examination of the chest usually demonstrates the characteristic signs of this condition.
    The affected lung may collapse all the way without causing much more than pain and shortness of breath as long as the other lung remains expanded. However, all but the smallest collapse should be reexpanded as soon as possible to avoid complications.
    Sometimes the tear in the lung results in a flap which lets air into the chest when the patient inhales, but will not let air escape back into the lung when he exhales. Air builds up in the damaged side and pushes the heart and large arteries and veins to the undamaged side. Blood return to the heart decreases, stops, and death results in a few minutes unless the pressure in the chest is relieved. This is a tension pneumothorax. It is very unusual in the absence of injury. The history of trauma and physical signs of pneumothorax make it unlikely that it will be mistaken for a cardiac problem. Treatment is immediate release of the built-up pressure with a needle in the chest and reexpansion of the lung as soon as possible.

Chapter Three

STRUCTURE AND FUNCTION—
HEART AND CHEST ORGANS

A. Summary

The fundamental unit of body structure is the cell. Cells are organized into functional units called organs. Examples of organs are the heart, brain, lungs, and kidneys.

Cells require energy to live and function. They get energy from the combination (reaction) of oxygen with compounds of carbon and hydrogen. Oxygen comes from air. The carbon-hydrogen compounds, which are among the things we call nutrients, are carbohydrates (sugars and starches), fats, and sometimes proteins. The waste products of the reaction are carbon dioxide and water. Blood takes oxygen and nutrients to the cells and carries carbon dioxide and water away from them. Blood is pumped by the heart.

The lungs are spongy masses of air sacs connected to the outside atmosphere by successively larger air passages. The walls of the sacs are made up of tiny blood vessels called capillaries. The capillaries have very thin walls through which oxygen can diffuse into blood and carbon dioxide and water can diffuse out of it. Lungs expand by the action of the ribs and the diaphragm, sucking in air. They contract by the action of their own elastic tissue, expelling air. The right heart pumps blood to the lungs through the pulmonary artery and its branches. The left heart receives blood from the lung through the pulmonary veins (fig. 3, p. 48).

Every organ of the body has its system of capillaries surrounding the cells. Oxygen and nutrients diffuse into the cells through the thin capillary walls; water and waste products from the cells diffuse in the opposite direction into the blood stream. The capillaries join to form larger and larger veins, finally becoming the superior vena cava and the inferior vena cava which empty into the right heart. The aorta carrying blood from the left heart branches into smaller and smaller arteries until it becomes a system of capillaries surrounding the body cells. Blood travels a closed circuit from body capillaries to right heart to lungs to left heart to body capillaries (fig. 2, p. 47).

The lungs and chest contents are separated from the abdomen by 2 dome shaped thin sheets of muscle called the left and right leaves of the diaphragm. Contraction of these muscle sheets when we breathe in flattens their dome shape; this in turn enlarges the chest cavity and expands the lungs.

The alimentary canal is the tube that carries nutrients from the mouth through the body. The part from the throat going down the middle of the chest in front of the backbone is called the esophagus. The esophagus joins the stomach just below the diaphragm. The dome of the stomach rises under the left leaf of the diaphragm and is a frequent source of the gas pains we feel in the chest. The stomach empties into the small intestine which in turn empties into the large intestine (colon). A loop of the large intestine coils under the left diaphragmatic leaf behind the stomach and may also be a source of chest pain.

Each side of the heart consists of 2 pumps, a thin-walled one called the atrium which leads directly to a thicker-walled one called the ventricle. The ventricles supply practically all the pumping power. At the entrance of each ventricle is a valve which, when the ventricle contracts, closes and prevents blood from flowing backward. The valves consist of thin flaps of tissue hanging from the walls of the ventricles. When the ventricles contract the flaps fill with blood and balloon out. Their free edges meet in the midline, shutting off flow back into the atrium.

Coming off the base of the aorta as it leaves the left ventricle are the right and left coronary arteries. These branch and spread over the heart, supplying it with blood. Atherosclerosis of these arteries is the central problem discussed in this book.

The electrical impulse that normally starts each heartbeat starts in a small clump of tissue in the right atrium called the SA node. The impulse then spreads successively through the atria and ventricles, causing them to contract in turn. Under unusual conditions any part of the heart muscle is capable of initiating an electrical impulse to start a heartbeat. A number of different types of abnormal beat patterns can occur; these are called dysrhythmias.

B. Why we need a heart

1. Cells and organs
The fundamental unit of body structure is the cell. Human body cells are too small to be seen without a microscope. There are many different types of cells; each type is specialized to perform one or a very few functions. For instance, muscle cells contract to provide motive power, nerve cells produce and transmit impulses, islet cells of the pancreas secrete insulin, and so on. Groups of different types of cells are organized into major body structures called organs, such as the heart, lungs, liver, and kidneys. Organs carry on the business of keeping us alive.

2. Energy production; nutrient and oxygen transport
Living, moving, thinking all require energy. Each cell gets its energy from a process like the burning of gasoline in an automobile engine; that is, the reaction of compounds of carbon and hydrogen with oxygen from air. The chief waste products of this reaction are carbon dioxide and water.

Food we eat is broken down to simpler substances in the stomach and intestine. These fragments are picked up by the circulating blood, taken to the liver for more processing to a form the cells can use, then delivered to the rest of the body. Blood also circulates through the lungs to pick up the oxygen required for oxidation, which is the name of the reaction that produces energy. Many additional substances such as vitamins, minerals, and the catalysts we call enzymes are necessary to make oxidation and chemical manufacture take place at body temperature. Some of these substances are present in foods; others are made at various places in the body.

Oxidation in an automobile engine is easier; all we need is a spark.

Blood is the circulating medium that picks all these things up, takes them where they need to go, and picks up waste products for proper disposal. The heart is the complex pump that circulates blood. The right side of the heart pumps blood to the lungs; the left side of the heart pumps blood to the rest of the body, including the heart itself. If the heart stops, the organs get no oxygen or nutrients and quit functioning. For example, if the brain is completely deprived of oxygen, consciousness is lost in about 15 seconds. The brain does not die that fast; just how long the brain can go without oxygen and not suffer irreversible damage is a subject of current investigation. Other organs do better than the brain. The heart can recover full function after an hour without oxygen provided (and this is a big provided) it is kept cool and not forced to pump blood. Without oxygen the energy supply of the heart is very limited; if it is forced to use this energy for pumping there is none left to keep it alive.

C. Organs of the chest

1. Lungs (fig. 1, p. 46)

The lungs are spongy masses of tiny air sacs called alveoli. The alveoli connect to successive generations of fewer and larger air passages and finally reach outside air at the vocal cords in the larynx (Adam's apple) in the middle of the throat. Each alveolus is surrounded by the body's smallest and thinnest blood vessels, the capillaries. The alveoli and capillaries are so small that we measure their size in microns. There are about 25,400 microns in each inch. Alveoli are about 75 to 300 microns and capillaries about 10 to 14 microns in diameter. The alveolar-capillary wall is less than $1/10$th micron thick. The lungs contain about 300 million alveoli. All this adds up to about 750 square feet of transfer surface to allow oxygen to diffuse into the body and carbon dioxide to diffuse out of it.

The whole mass of the lungs is crisscrossed with elastic fibers so that the lungs tend to collapse into small balls with no air unless they are kept expanded by adhesion of their surfaces to the inner chest walls. The lungs and chest walls stick together by means of a thin layer of liquid, just as 2 flat glass plates can be held together by a thin layer of water between them. The bottom surface of the lung sticks to the diaphragm in the same way. During inspiration (breathing in) the dome of the diaphragm flattens and the normally downslanting bucket-handles of the ribs assume a more nearly horizontal position. These actions increase the volume of the chest cavity, causing air to flow into the lungs. During expiration (breathing out) the diaphragm and the muscles between the ribs relax. The elastic fibers in the lungs cause them to shrink, expelling air.

2. Blood vessels in the chest (figs. 1-3, pp. 46-48)

Blood from the capillary beds of the head, arms, and chest (except the lungs) is picked up by a network of veins which join in a succession of larger and fewer vessels to form the superior vena cava. The superior vena cava empties into the right atrium. Similarly, the capillary beds of the legs, pelvis, and abdomen connect by a network of veins to the inferior vena cava which also empties into the right atrium. Blood from the right atrium flows into the right ventricle, which in turn pumps it to the lungs through the pulmonary artery. The main pulmonary artery splits into the right and left pulmonary arteries which supply their respective lungs. They do this by breaking up into smaller and smaller branches, finally forming the pulmonary capillary beds. The capillaries reform into the pulmonary veins which connect to the left atrium. From there blood flows into the left ventricle which pumps it into the aorta. The aorta branches to supply the capillary beds of all the tissues of the body.

3. Pericardium

The heart hangs free in the chest, attached to the major blood vessels. It is suspended in a sac of fibrous tissue called the pericardium. Normally the sac contains nearly 2 ounces of fluid which serves as a lubricant for the very active motion of the heart. There is not room in the sac for much more than this; if as little as 6 to 8 more ounces of fluid collects in the sac rapidly it may crowd the heart, not allowing it to fill properly. Such a collection, called a pericardial effusion, may result from inflammation, trauma, or disease. A tear in the heart or blood vessel inside the pericardium may allow a blood leak with the same result. If the fluid collects slowly the pericardium can stretch to accommodate much more than

8 ounces. Inflammation of the pericardium can cause pain; this will be discussed in chapter IV.

4. Esophagus, stomach, intestine, and diaphragm (fig. 1, p. 46)
The esophagus lies behind the heart and lungs at the back of the chest in the midline. It is the tube that carries food from the throat to the stomach. Acid from the stomach sometimes gets into the esophagus and causes the sensation we call "heartburn". Heartburn has nothing to do with the heart. The esophagus normally moves food by waves of muscular contraction followed by waves of relaxation. The waves start at the throat and push food into the stomach. The process is called peristalsis; it is initiated by swallowing. Sometimes peristalsis becomes disordered and a ring of contraction persists in one area. This is spasm as we have previously defined that term (chapter I). Sometimes spasm can be relieved by swallowing medicine and sometimes not. The pain of esophageal spasm may be difficult to distinguish from cardiac pain.

As it leaves the chest the esophagus joins the stomach. The stomach in turn empties into the intestine where food is further broken down and absorbed. The intestines are coiled and folded; the stomach and parts of the intestine are found in the left upper part of the abdomen where they are separated from the heart, left lung, and other chest contents by the thin sheet of muscle we call the left diaphragm. The left diaphragm is dome shaped; its central part, with the stomach and intestine under it, may rise as high as the nipple line in the center of the left chest. Pockets of air or gas may form in the stomach or intestine, press on the diaphragm, and cause chest pain. Such pockets cannot press on the heart or cause any heart problems.

5. Nerve supply; site of origin of pain
There are "nerves" and then there are nerves. By "nerves" people frequently mean emotional problems such as a "nervous breakdown".

The nerves we are talking about are different. They are long branching bundles of very thin fibers much like miniature telephone cables. They connect the various parts of the body to the brain and spinal cord and have much the same function as telephone cables; they carry orders from the brain

42

to the body and carry information (including pain sensation) from the body to the brain.

The heart, diaphragm, most of the other organs we have mentioned, and parts of the left arm get their nerve supply from the same segments of the spinal cord. Regardless of which of these structures the pain comes from, it is often felt in the left chest and left arm. As a result, location of pain is not much help in deciding its origin. In particular, pain in the chest going down the left arm is not necessarily cardiac; it may be coming from the esophagus, diaphragm, chest wall muscles, pleura, or other structures.

Figure 1, p. 46, shows the left chest and abdomen. The crowding and overlapping of structures are obvious causes of the difficulty we sometimes have in pinning down the origin of pain.

6. The heart; structure and function (figs. 3-7, pp. 48-52)

We said earlier that the right heart pumps blood from the body to the lungs and the left heart pumps blood from the lungs to the body. Each side of the heart consists of 2 pumps, the atrium and ventricle, connected one after the other (in series), making 4 pumps for the whole heart. Each pump is a sac whose walls are mainly made of layers of a special kind of muscle cell (myocardial cells). Pump action consists of the muscle cells contracting in a carefully coordinated manner to squeeze blood out of the sac, followed by relaxation of the cells to allow the sacs to fill with blood.

The first or upper sac on each side, the atrium, is very thin-walled. It contracts slightly before the second sac, the ventricle, does, and serves chiefly to increase ventricular filling. The ventricles are much thicker-walled than the atria and do practically all the work of pumping. The left ventricle is thicker-walled than the right. It has to pump against a higher pressure; the blood pressure in the aorta is normally much higher than that in the pulmonary artery.

7. The heartbeat; valves

Every heartbeat (60 to 80 times a minute at rest, up to 180 or more times a minute with strenuous exercise or excitement) consists of 2 phases: a relaxation phase, diastole, during which the ventricles fill, and a contraction phase, systole, during which the ventricles empty. There has to be some mechanism to keep blood from flowing backward. This is provided by the valves of the heart, aorta, and pulmonary artery. A valve is anything that serves to control the flow of fluid (liquid or gas). An ordinary water faucet is a valve, but much different in operating principle from the valves of the heart.

Heart valves (figs. 5-6, pp. 50-51) may be visualized by imagining 2 parachutes attached by parts of their rims to opposite sides of the inside wall of a pipe. Fluid flowing from the convex (bulge toward you) to the concave (bulge away from you) side of the chutes collapses them against the wall of the pipe so they do not obstruct flow. Any attempt to force fluid to flow in the opposite direction, from concave to convex side, immediately fills out the chutes. Their free edges meet in the middle of the pipe and the billowed out chutes completely stop the flow of fluid. We attach the free edges of the chutes to the walls of the pipe on their concave sides to keep these edges from being forced past each other.

The atria have no valves. At the entrance to the right ventricle there is a valve with 3 parachutes (called cusps or leaflets) named the tricuspid valve. At the entrance to the left ventricle there is a valve with 2 cusps called the mitral valve. The strands of tissue attaching the free edges of these valve cusps to the walls of the ventricles are called chordae tendineae. They attach to muscular projections from the inside walls of the ventricles; the projections are called papillary muscles. The aorta and pulmonary artery each have a valve where they join the left and right ventricles respectively. These valves have 3 cusps, are smaller than the mitral and tricuspid valves, and have no chordae tendineae.

8. Coronary arteries; the blood supply to the heart
   (fig. 4, p. 49)

Blood for the heart is furnished by the right and left coronary arteries. These originate as holes (the coronary ostia) in the walls of the aorta inside the pockets of 2 of the 3 cusps of the aortic valve. The arteries branch, spread over the surface of the heart, and penetrate its substance. The branches interconnect with each other in a highly variable way; the interconnections are collectively called the collateral circulation. The collateral circulation becomes very important as a secondary source of blood for the part of the heart involved when a coronary branch is partly or totally blocked.

9. The electrical system; cardiac rhythm

Normally the electrical impulse starting each heartbeat originates in a small area in the inner wall of the right atrium called the sinoatrial (SA) node. From the SA node the impulse spreads through both atria, causing them to contract. In the normal heart conduction between the atria and ventricles is blocked everywhere except at one small spot called the atrioventricular or AV node. Conduction is slightly delayed at the AV node. The impulse then passes through the node into a bundle of fibers in the ventricle called the bundle of His. This bundle breaks up into 3 branches (the bundle branches) which then form a network of conducting fibers (the Purkinje network) spreading through both ventricles.

Changes in heartbeat pattern such as fast beating, slow beating, extra beats, or irregular beats may be the result of changes anywhere in the heart but frequently result from problems in the conduction system. Altered beat patterns are called dysrhythmias. Sometimes a dysrhythmia is an indication of disease, sometimes not. Some of the dysrhythmias most disturbing to people who have them are totally harmless, as for instance the extra beats of our patient #5 (chapter I). However, dysrhythmias may at times be the first or only sign of ischemic heart disease. We will discuss them more in the section on electrocardiography (chapter VII).

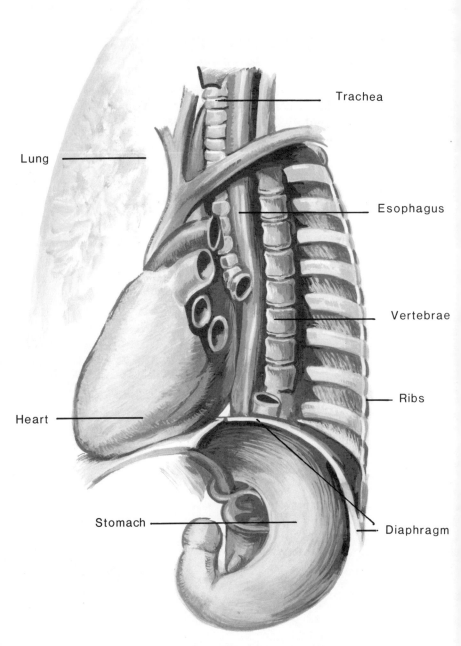

Trachea

Lung

Esophagus

Vertebrae

Ribs

Heart

Stomach

Diaphragm

LEFT SIDE OF CHEST
AND UPPER ABDOMEN

Fig. 1

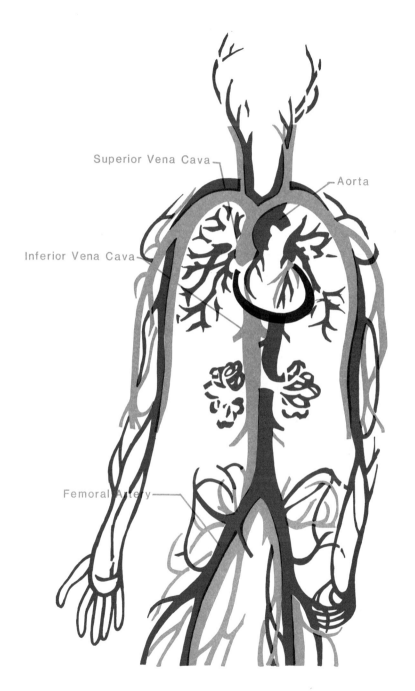

Superior Vena Cava

Aorta

Inferior Vena Cava

Femoral Artery

Body Circulation

47   **Fig. 2**

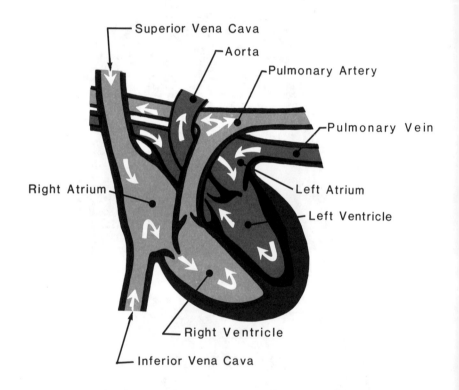

Superior Vena Cava

Aorta

Pulmonary Artery

Pulmonary Vein

Right Atrium

Left Atrium

Left Ventricle

Right Ventricle

Inferior Vena Cava

Fig. 3

48

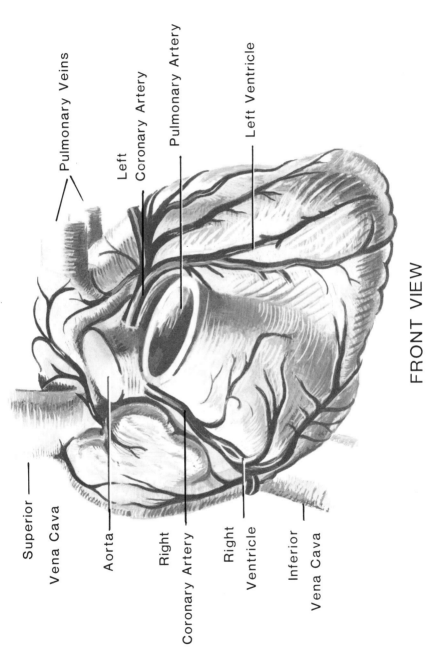

Superior Vena Cava

Pulmonary Veins

Left Coronary Artery

Aorta

Right Coronary Artery

Pulmonary Artery

Right Ventricle

Left Ventricle

Inferior Vena Cava

FRONT VIEW

Fig. 4

49

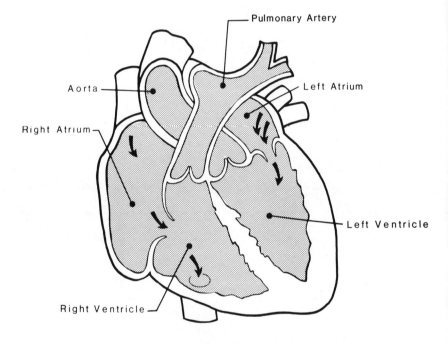

Pulmonary Artery

Aorta

Right Atrium

Left Atrium

Left Ventricle

Right Ventricle

Diastole

Fig. 5

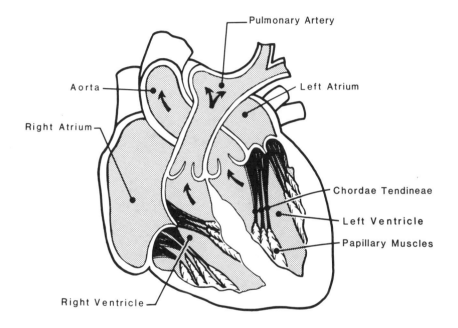

Pulmonary Artery

Aorta

Left Atrium

Right Atrium

Chordae Tendineae

Left Ventricle

Papillary Muscles

Right Ventricle

Systole

Fig. 6

51

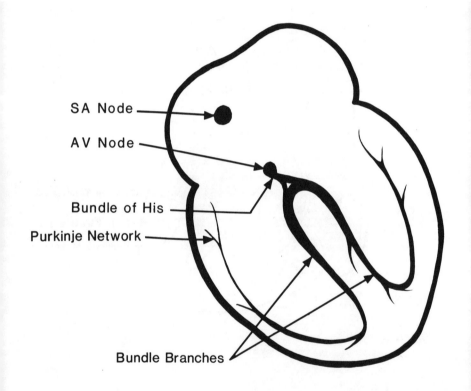

SA Node

AV Node

Bundle of His

Purkinje Network

Bundle Branches

Fig. 7

Chapter Four

NON-CARDIAC CHEST PAIN

A. Summary

Nearly all the non-cardiac structures of the chest wall and chest interior can produce pain. Except for problems with the aorta, pulmonary artery, and sudden severe lung collapse, this pain is very rarely associated with the threat of sudden death. The non-cardiac structures in and near the chest which are most likely to cause pain are skin and tissue under it, muscles, ribs, inner lining of the chest wall (parietal pleura), sac containing the heart (pericardium), esophagus, stomach, intestines, and diaphragm.

Skin pain is usually caused by infection, injury, or nerve irritation. The part involved is frequently tender and the pain bright and well localized. Local warmth and redness may indicate an infection.

Pain from muscles and ribs comes mainly from exercise or trauma. The pain is usually made worse by local pressure or deep breathing. Pain may not show up for 2 or 3 days after the strain or exercise causing it. Ribs may be cracked by injury, coughing, laughing, hugging, or sneezing; the cause of a rib fracture may not be obvious. A rib fracture may not be evident on x-ray for 10 to 14 days after the injury.

Neurocirculatory asthenia is an especially troublesome form of chest pain. It has a number of other names as well. Although the pain is associated with emotional tension, the mechanism for its production is not known. Since it occurs on the left side in tense people and shows up over and over again, it is usually hard to convince patients that it does not come from the heart. It does not. The pain is physically harmless and is not an indication of organic disease.

The inner lining of the chest wall (parietal pleura) is very pain sensitive. Pain from this structure is called pleurisy. Although the lung and its covering (visceral pleura) are not pain sensitive, irritation from a lung infection or blood clot may spread to the inner chest wall covering and cause pain. The pain is almost always sharp and is made worse by breathing.

The heart hangs free in a sac called the pericardium. The sac sometimes becomes inflamed and painful, a condition called pericarditis. The pain is usually sharp and steady but may be dull or aching. It is frequently made worse by lying down and better by sitting up and leaning forward.

The esophagus is the food tube from the mouth to the stomach; it passes through the chest. Pain from this structure is usually recognized as the familiar heartburn or indigestion. It may however show up as a sudden severe sharp pain or a dull ache which responds poorly to the usual indigestion medicines. Careful testing and examination may at times be required to distinguish this pain from heart pain.

The left diaphragm and the stomach and large intestine under it are frequent sources of chest pain. This is usually but not always recognized as "gas pain". The pain is often sharp or cramping; even if it is dull it may be identified by the way it changes with shifting intestinal gas.

Tumors sometimes cause pain by pressure on or invasion of chest structures. This is usually a late sign; the presence of a tumor at this stage is commonly easy to demonstrate.

B. Introduction

If we look at our entire population, there are many more episodes of non-cardiac than cardiac chest pain each year. Most non-cardiac pain is recognized as not being a serious health threat and is more or less ignored. If the pain is recurrent or persistent it may indicate a definite disease process. Sometimes the disease is minor, sometimes serious.

Minor or serious, these diseases vary from ischemic heart disease in one very important way. With the few exceptions described in chapter II, they are very rarely associated with the threat of sudden death. Non-cardiac chest pain has no direct effect on the heart. It may however become a form of stress which increases cardiac work and irritability. There is no evidence that this bothers a normal heart in any way; it may aggravate cardiac problems which are already present.

The structures we are going to discuss are the most important but not the only ones involved in the production of non-cardiac chest pain. They are skin and underlying tissue, muscles of the chest and arm, ribs and the muscles between them, inside lining of the chest wall (parietal pleura), lungs, sac containing the heart (pericardium), food tube (esophagus), leaf of muscle separating lungs from stomach (diaphragm), and stomach and intestines (chapter III).

C. Skin and subcutaneous tissue

Pain in the skin and tissue under it is usually caused by infection, injury, or nerve irritation. Most of the time the pain is well localized. The area is frequently tender.

Infections may be due to germs or viruses. Shingles (herpes zoster) deserves special mention. It is an infection of skin, skin nerves, and nerve roots caused by the same virus that causes chicken pox. The pain may be sharp, burning, or aching, or any combination of these. If the nerves supplying the chest wall are affected, the pain may be thought to be coming from the heart. Careful examination usually makes it evident that the pain is in the skin. At first the skin may look completely normal; however, at some time in the course of the illness the patient breaks out with one or more patches of red rash and blisters along the course of the involved nerve. The rash is characteristic and usually establishes the cause of the pain. Sometimes older people are left with a chronic nagging ache after the rash clears. There is no treatment that is dramatically effective; some medicines now in use seem to shorten the course of the illness and make it milder.

Skin infections caused by germs usually show local redness, tenderness, and swelling; pain from them is rarely confused with that from deeper structures. These infections are treated with antibiotics and, if pus is present, surgical drainage.

D. Chest muscles and ribs

Exercise and injury are common causes of chest pain (patient #4, chapter I). Pain from muscle strain may show up as late as 3 or 4 days after the activity causing it. Chronic strain from such things as poor posture while typing, filing in awkward positions, and improper lifting can cause chest and left arm pain. Crowding of the nerves as they leave the neck or armpit sometimes causes similar pain.

This pain comes from muscles or nerves. It may take persistent questioning and examination to establish the cause, but tenderness of the muscles and/or aggravation of the pain by some specific movements will usually be distinctive characteristics. There is no connection with or effect of any kind on the heart; it is surprising how difficult it is to convince some patients of this, even though the muscular origin is plainly demonstrated to them.

Pain may of course be caused by rib fractures or bruises. This cause is easy to spot if there has been a recognized injury; however, ribs may be broken by coughing, sneezing, laughing, hugging, or straining. The patient may have forgotten the incident entirely, especially if he had a few drinks. Tenderness at the fracture site and pain with breathing ordinarily make the cause of the pain easy to identify. X-rays usually show the break but can be misleading; it may take as many as 2 weeks for evidence of fracture to appear on the films.

Inflammation of rib cartilage next to the sternum (breastbone) just to either side of the midline of the chest is also a fairly common cause of pain. The condition is called Tietze's syndrome. The pain may or may not be made worse by breathing or motion, but tenderness of the ribs at the front of the chest is almost always present. Sometimes an enlarged knob can be felt at the end of the rib near the sternum. No one knows the cause. X-rays are required to rule out other problems. It is not progressive, not a threat to health, and causes no trouble but pain. Treatment is heat and pain medication. Local injections can be used if the trouble persists.

The muscles of the chest wall between the ribs are very sensitive to pain. Either aching or sharp stabbing pain may develop in these muscles, usually as a result of exercise.

E. "Neurocirculatory asthenia," "periapical fatigue"

Patient #5 (chapter I) provides an example of a common and disconcerting type of chest pain. It has been called "soldier's heart," "neurasthenia," "Da Costa's syndrome," and the 2 names above among other things. All these names are meaningless; they only emphasize the fact that we do not understand the mechanism of production of the pain. It is on the left side of the chest and may go down the left arm. It may be sharp or aching; it is rarely described as pressure like. The chest wall is usually tender. Breathing may or may not make the pain worse.

It frequently lasts hours, days, or weeks, getting better and worse during the period. The pain is not made worse by exercise the patient enjoys; often it gets better or disappears when the patient becomes preoccupied with physical exertion.

The pain is strongly related to emotional tension. It may be only loosely or not at all connected to any specific episode of stress, but the patient is tense and anxious. It must be emphasized that the pain is real; it is in the patient's chest, not his head. Depending on how the patient reacts, the pain may be anything from a mild nuisance to incapacitating.

Treatment is often difficult. The patient may partly or completely reject the idea that the pain is emotionally conditioned. He gets a cardiac workup, sometimes more than one, including electrocardiograms, monitors, stress tests, echocardiogram, and possibly angiography (chapter VII). Any deviation from the usual, such as our patient #5's premature beats, is seized on as evidence that the pain is cardiac. It is not. It has nothing to do with the heart. The pain is not a threat to life or physical well being and is not associated with any increased risk of sudden death. Other illnesses, including heart diseases, may of course occur in patients with this problem. If so, they are treated just as if the pain were not present. Some pain clinics are having success in treating this disorder with combinations of physical measures and counselling.

F. Pleurisy

The parietal pleura is the inside lining of the chest wall; the visceral pleura is the outer covering of the lung. They are in contact with each other through a thin layer of liquid (chapter III). The parietal pleura is pain sensitive, the visceral pleura and lung are not. However, lung problems frequently affect the parietal pleura, causing pain. Usually the pain results from infection, trauma, pneumothorax, or pulmonary embolism (chapter II). It is generally sharp and made worse by breathing; it goes by the familiar name of pleurisy. Seriousness of the problem depends on the underlying cause. This is another situation where severity of the pain has very little connection with the gravity of the illness. Very painful viral infections may clear completely in a few days with no treatment. On the other hand, pneumonia involving large amounts of lung tissue may cause little pain. Treatment must be directed at the responsible condition.

G. Pericardium
The heart hangs loosely in a thin tough sac called the pericardium. Inflammation of the pericardium is called pericarditis; it may be due to many different causes. The associated pain may be sharp or aching; it is usually steady but may vary with breathing. Unlike the pain of myocardial infarction, it often changes with position. It is usually made worse by lying down and is somewhat relieved by sitting up and leaning forward. It is not related to effort and is not relieved by nitroglycerin or similar medications. A rub or scratching sound may be heard with each heartbeat. There are often characteristic electrocardiographic changes. If fluid collects in the pericardial sac, it may be evident on the echocardiogram (chapter VII).

Treatment depends on the cause. It may involve pain medication, steroids, antibiotics, drainage of fluid, correction of problems in other organs, or surgical removal of the pericardium.

H. Esophagus
This is the food tube from the throat to the stomach. It is in the midline at the rear of the chest. The wall of the esophagus contains the same special type of muscle (called smooth muscle, from its microscopic characteristics) that is found in the walls of arteries. Like arteries, the esophagus can go into spasm. Causes of pain and spasm may be anything from stomach acid to irritating foods or chemicals (including alcohol) to emotional stress. Almost everyone at one time or another has had the familiar sensation of heartburn or indigestion from one of these causes. Sometimes, however, esophageal pain is a dull ache under the sternum, much like the pain of ischemic heart disease; it may go to the left arm as well. To add to the confusion, relief is often

obtained from nitroglycerin under the tongue; nitroglycerin relaxes smooth muscle spasm in the esophagus as well as in arteries. Swallowing would be expected to aggravate the pain but often does not. The discomfort may last hours to days; sometimes patients have to be hospitalized for observation and testing to be sure they do not have some form of cardiac ischemia.

Esophageal problems are treated with medicines whose purpose is to prevent acid reflux, react with the acid, and decrease acid production and spasm. In unusual cases surgery may be necessary.

I. Diaphragm, stomach, intestines

The left diaphragm is a thin leaf of connective tissue and muscle which separates the chest from the abdomen on the left side. The bottom of the left lung and heart are in contact with its upper surface; stomach and intestines are immediately underneath it. The center of the left diaphragm is supplied by some of the same nerves that supply the left arm; its outer part has the same nerve supply as the left chest wall. The diaphragm is very sensitive; bubbles in the stomach or intestine may cause pain in those structures or by pressure on the diaphragm. The pain may be sharp or dull. It may be felt in the chest, left arm, or both. Frequently the pain moves or changes with stomach or intestinal burbling; this immediately pinpoints its source. There is no way gas in the stomach or intestine can press on the heart. However, on rare occasions the pain of ischemic heart disease may be felt in the upper abdomen.

Sometimes there is a defect in the left diaphragm called a hiatus hernia, through which stomach or intestine can push into the chest. While these misplaced organs can cause pain, especially when the person lies down, they do not push on the heart or cause cardiac problems.

Treatment, if it is necessary, is much the same as that for esophageal pain. Surgery may sometimes be needed for hiatus hernia.

J. Tumors

Benign tumors or cancers may involve any chest structure and cause pain. A tumor may appear as a lump in a rib or the chest wall. The pain is usually a nagging ache, at least to start with, and is rarely thought to have a cardiac origin.

Tumors may cause sudden death by eroding into a blood vessel and causing massive bleeding or by shutting off the air supply to the lungs. These are generally late effects; the presence of the tumor has usually been recognized before they occur.

Chapter Five

STATISTICS, TESTS, TREATMENTS, AND MEDICAL "PROOF"

A. Summary

Because of the large number of factors that influence them, human responses vary greatly. This is true in medicine as in every other field of human activity. As a result, we have no perfect tests and no 100% effective medicines or procedures. Reasons for changes in health, both in individuals and in large populations, are often difficult to evaluate.

Statistics is the science of imperfect results and inadequate information. By statistical means we attempt to decide how good a test or medicine is and to establish the importance of cause and effect relationships in the presence of complicating factors.

The 2 simplest measures of test quality are sensitivity and specificity. Sensitivity is the percent of instances a test is positive when it should be positive; specificity is the percent of instances a test is negative when it should be negative. For example, if we test 100 people who should all have positive results and only 90 do, the test is 90% sensitive. If we test 100 people and all should have negative results but only 95 do, the test is 95% specific.

Testing for diseases of low occurrence rate (low incidence) in large populations poses special problems; even very good tests give disappointingly low yields of useful information. This situation arises in attempting to test for ischemic heart disease in the general population.

There are also a number of problems in attempting to design and carry out tests of drugs and procedures. The double blind study has been developed in an attempt to control some of these difficulties. When it can be performed properly it is very valuable; even with this study there are many pitfalls to be guarded against.

Epidemiologic investigations are those in which the researcher gathers and attempts to interpret information on changes in free living populations where there are no imposed experimental conditions. Such studies have been done in attempts to explain the recorded 39% drop in death rate from ischemic heart disease in the past 20 years. As is common in situations of this kind, there has been a great deal of argument on the interpretation of results.

All our studies are done in an attempt to give us information on risk versus benefit for any action we plan to take or not take. In most cases the indicated decision is clearcut; sometimes choices can be difficult.

B. Introduction

When we do something or take something, how do we know that we are doing ourselves more good than harm? When a medical test is performed, how do we know that it is giving us reliable information? Are the lifestyle changes we see all around us really of any use in preventing ischemic heart disease?

Answers to these questions are far from obvious. If someone is sick, takes medicine, and gets well there is no way to tell in any one instance that the medicine was responsible. We must observe a number of cases. Even with the best medicines there are treatment failures. If we get more good results with the medicine than without, we still have to decide whether they were related to the medicine, to chance, to patient selection, or to other factors we have not recognized. The same problems arise when we try to develop new tests. No test is perfect. If a test looks useful, we have to be as sure as we can that it is the test and not just something else making it look good.

None of our questions, tests, medicines, or procedures is

perfect. If not, how good are they? New ones are constantly being developed. We would like to use the most effective (and if possible the simplest and cheapest) ones available. How do we judge?

C. Sensitivity and specificity

Evaluation of tests may not be easy but is usually fairly straightforward. First we decide how to establish that a particular disease is present. This may mean exhaustive and complicated testing that is not possible on a routine basis but is necessary for research purposes. One way or another we throw out any doubtful cases. Then we apply the test to people who have the illness and see what percent are positive. This is the sensitivity of the test. We also apply the test to a large number of people who do not have the illness and see what percent are negative. This is the specificity of the test.

To restate the definitions, sensitivity is the ratio of test positives to total people with the disease; specificity is the ratio of test negatives to people without the disease. A perfect test would be 100% sensitive and 100% specific. Practically speaking, we have no perfect tests. Real people and real diseases are just too variable. The numbers provide a good means of comparing tests. They do not compare cost, availability, convenience, time, or safety, any one of which rather than sensitivity or specificity may be the governing consideration in deciding if a test will be used.

To get better results we use more tests. For example, we may consider the medical history a test. Its actual sensitivity will vary with the disease, the patient, and the doctor, but for illustration let us use 90%. This means the test will miss 10 patients out of 100. If we apply a second independent test that is also 90% sensitive it will pick up 9 of the remaining 10; the combined tests will have a sensitivity of 99% and will miss only one out of 100.

In practice we cannot attach concrete numbers to many of our observations. We use history, examinations, and tests over a period of time until we have established the diagnosis to our satisfaction.

D. Small groups in large populations

There is another catch when we apply tests for diseases with small numbers of cases in large populations. The following example gets a little involved but is of great practical importance.

We know that 1% of the 35 million men in the U.S. between the ages of 35 and 60 will develop ischemic heart disease each year. That is 350,000 men. We also know that 13% of this group, or about 45,000, will have cardiac arrests and another 147,000 will have myocardial infarctions. We want to find the 350,000 men so we can start treatment and do our best to head off the disaster facing 192,000 of them.

Suppose we develop a test that will predict which of our 35 million men will be affected, and suppose that the test is 95% sensitive and 95% specific. 95%-95% figures are good for any medical test; for one like we are dreaming about that could be applied to 35 million people they would be remarkable. But let us suppose anyway. We pick up 332,000 or 95% of the 350,000 who are going to develop ischemic heart disease. We miss about 18,000 but that is better than missing 350,000. Unfortunately, our test is also going to be positive for 5% of the remaining 34,650,000 or 1,732,000 who do not have ischemic heart disease (our false positives). We would be treating 1,732,000 who did not need it as well as 332,000 who did. This is a batting average of 16% and is not practical for long term interventions like those required for ischemic heart disease.

The problem is an unavoidable consequence of using tests, even very good ones, for diseases of low incidence. A solution is to apply a second test to our positives. If we can find a second 95%-95% test completely independent of the first and use it on all our positives, we would wind up with 316,000 true positives and 87,000 false positives. We lose an additional 17,000 people we should be treating, but we are not treating 1,600,000 people we should not be. With further testing we keep losing people who need treatment but sooner or later get to what we decide is an acceptably low false positive number.

So we almost always use multiple tests. No matter how many tests we use, we can never be 100% sure. We cannot use the words "never" and "always" about our results. We have to settle for "usually" and "rarely" and so on.

This difficulty with diseases of low incidence results from testing limitations and does not occur in the care of individual patients for 2 reasons. First, every question we ask or examination we do on the patient is a test in the sense in which we are using the word. We can perform a great number of these in a short time when we are working on a one to one basis. Second, implied in the procedures on large numbers of patients is the fact that we do not retest negatives. This is not true of the individual patient. We continue with him as long as we like, no matter what category a particular test puts him in. As a result, while we can still never be 100% certain, we can as a practical matter make our margin of error extremely small.

E. Treatment and prevention
Our difficulties increase by leaps and bounds when it comes to evaluating treatment and prevention measures. Diseases vary greatly in their natural histories; they may get worse, stay the same, or get better in an unpredictable way on no treatment. This is especially true of diseases like atherosclerosis and its complications where the process usually covers many years.

Furthermore, many people respond to any new treatment by feeling better. This is especially likely if they have a good relationship with an optimistic doctor. The patient may feel better for a time while his disease is getting worse. He could be using a useless medication instead of a useful one, with disastrous results down the line.

To get around most of these problems the double blind study and its variations have been adopted as the standard for testing medical procedures and treatments. If, for example, we want to evaluate a new medicine for treating a disease, we gather as large a group of people with the disease as we can. We then randomly assign every patient to one of 2 subgroups. If our randomization process has been adequate (and this can be a problem) the 2 subgroups should be very close to the same in every respect that might count (age, sex, severity of disease, and so on). One group we treat with the medicine; the other group gets an inert material (called a placebo) disguised to look, smell, taste, and feel as much like the medicine as possible. Neither the patient (single blind) nor the doctor (double blind) giving the materials and evaluating the results knows which is medicine and which is placebo. Alternatively, another medicine may be used in place of the placebo.

Even when they can be used, such studies still may have many problems. How much difference in result is a real difference as opposed to one that might be due purely to chance? Arbitrarily (meaning the figure was picked as being "reasonable") it has been widely accepted that a difference that would occur by chance one time in 20 or less is "real", or in fancier terms "statistically significant". The reader will have to consult a statistics book to see how the one in 20 is calculated. Use of this standard does not mean that we cannot be wrong in attaching significance or lack of it to our results. It just means we should be wrong one time in 20 or less on the average.

There are more possible difficulties. How do we know that our group of patients is truly representative of all patients with the disease? Is the group large enough? Are our subgroups comparable? Are our evaluation methods for the progress of the disease good enough? Have we sufficiently disguised our placebo? How much and how long should we test for side effects? Are the patients taking the medicine like they are supposed to? This compliance problem really becomes severe in prevention trials where we are often asking groups of free living healthy people to change their living patterns, sometimes for years, to see if the change will keep them from getting a disease.

Doctors are aware of these and other confounding problems that can occur even in well designed studies. They are understandably skeptical of front page miracle cures that have not gone through a rigorous evaluation.

F. Epidemiologic investigations

So far we have talked about tests and experiments. We are also interested in the changes occurring in people who are not part of any experiment; we call these free living populations.

For instance, Japanese men have more ischemic heart disease when they move from Japan to the U.S. Japanese men also eat more fat, especially saturated fat, when they move from Japan to the U.S.. Is this cause and effect?

Obviously, changing countries involves much more than a change in fat intake. There are other dietary and life-style changes that could conceivably have a big influence on the development of atherosclerosis.

Since we have no control over our subjects, all we can do is gather as much detailed information as possible. We then use an assortment of statistical methods to try to determine what factors are important. The results are often not easy to interpret. We will see this in chapter IX when we discuss the reasons for the big drop in the ischemic heart disease death rate in the U.S. in the past 20 years.

G. Risks versus benefit

All our tests and evaluations finally boil down to one evaluation; we assemble all the information we can and make a risk versus benefit judgment concerning everything we do or plan to do.

For example, we usually consider taking a medical history a risk-free procedure we are willing to use on everyone. Even this is not entirely true. If a patient has an obvious myocardial infarction we should not be asking about his grandmother's health; we had better get started on treatment immediately. At other times taking a detailed medical history may be the most important procedure we can institute.

Similarly, an electrocardiogram, which just measures electrical currents from the heart, involves only the risk that there is something more important we should be doing. When we get to procedures like the stress test and coronary angiography (chapter VII) the situation changes. The procedures themselves involve a small but definite risk. We need to be sure that what we expect to learn is worth that risk.

There is, also, no such thing as a risk-free medication or surgical procedure. Every dose of medicine or operation carries with it the risk of bad effects. Sometimes the risk is slight, sometimes it is appreciable, but is must always be considered.

Chapter Six

MITRAL VALVE PROLAPSE

A. Summary

A valve is by definition something which controls the flow of fluid. The mitral valve consists of 2 thin flaps of tissue at the entrance to the left ventricle (fig. 6, p. 51). When the left ventricle contracts, these flaps normally come together to close its entrance and keep blood from flowing backward into the atrium. In most people the domes of the closed valve do not bulge beyond the ring which marks the border between the left atrium and the left ventricle (figs 8-9, pp. 74-75).

Mitral valve prolapse (abbreviated MVP) is the bulging of one or both leaflets of the mitral valve into the left atrium when the left ventricle contracts. It has been found in anywhere from 2% to 28% of various groups of adults examined in the general population—2% in elderly males, 28% in grossly underweight young females. A conservative estimate is that at least 5 million people in the U.S. have mitral valve prolapse. There are a number of possible causes. In the great majority of instances it is a normal variation; as such it is not connected with any threat to life or health, present or future. Sometimes, however, MVP indicates an underlying disease which may be a serious problem. Rarely, sudden death occurs in people with these diseases. Even in these cases, there is no evidence that the prolapse is the cause of death; people with these same diseases who do not have MVP may also die suddenly.

There is no statistical evidence of association between MVP and chest pain. In populations studied, just as great a percent of people without MVP as with MVP have chest pain.

However, MVP may be a marker for heart disease. As with other findings such as murmurs, cardiac irregularities, and chest pain itself, MVP should always be carefully evaluated by a competent physician to determine whether or not heart disease is present.

B. MVP—what is it

Chapter III discusses heart and heart valve structures and function. We are going to go over the subject here as it relates to MVP.

The heart consists of 4 chambers, the right and left atria and the right and left ventricles (fig. 3, p. 48). Blood travels successively to the body, right atrium, right ventricle, lungs, left atrium, left ventricle, then back to the body. The pumps that keep the blood circulating are the right and left ventricles. These are sacs of muscle. They pump by first relaxing, allowing themselves to be filled with blood. This stage of the process is called diastole. The muscle fibers in the walls then contract, shrinking the sacs and forcing blood out. This stage is called systole.

To keep blood from flowing backward there is a valve in each ventricle where it joins the atrium. The one in the left ventricle is called the mitral valve. It consists of 2 flexible leaflets (called cusps) attached to the inner rim of the left ventricular opening. During relaxation (diastole) the leaflets flatten near the ventricular walls, allowing blood to flow freely. When contraction (systole) starts, the leaflets fill with blood and balloon out. Their edges meet and effectively seal the opening into the atrium. The free edges of the leaflets are attached to projections (called papillary muscles) from the inner walls of the ventricle. This arrangement keeps the valve edges from blowing past each other during systole.

In most individuals no part of a valve leaflet protrudes into the atrium at any time during the cardiac cycle. In some people, however, part of a leaflet bulges past the ventricular opening at some time during systole. This is MVP (figs. 8-9, pp. 74-75).

C. Diagnosis of MVP—echocardiography

A special type of click, sometimes accompanied by a murmur, has been considered to be characteristic of MVP. The reported reliability of these findings has varied from study to study.

Currently, the presence of MVP is almost always established by ultrasound examination (chapter VII). Ultrasound is sound of much higher pitch than can be heard by the human ear. The sound echoes from boundaries between materials of different densities, especially boundaries between liquids and solids. The surfaces of the mitral valves are such boundaries. Since the speed of the sound and the time of the sound-echo round trip can be measured accurately, the location of any part of the mitral valve can be established precisely at any instant. Any bulging of any part of the valve into the atrium can be pinpointed to within 2 millimeters (about 1/10th of an inch) or less. This type of study is called echocardiography. Since it uses only sound waves, it has no known bad effects. However, its proper performance and interpretation require skill and experience.

D. Incidence of MVP—who has it

The best way to find out how much MVP is present in the general population and what problems are associated with it is to study large unselected groups of people—that is, unselected with respect to anything that might have the slightest bearing on their cardiovascular status.

Reported figures vary quite a bit. There is general agreement that the condition occurs most often in young women. 4 to 17% of women in their 20's and 30's have been found to have MVP. Some of this variability in reported rates probably results from differences in echocardiographic technique and the criteria used for the diagnosis. On the other hand, there is no doubt much true variation from group to group. One reason for the differences in study results is the large range of weights in women subjects. A recent study found that 9 out of 26 (28%) of grossly underweight young women with anorexia nervosa had MVP. When they gained weight under treatment, 7 (all that could be checked; 2 were lost to follow-up) lost their MVP. Later still, 3 of these women lost weight again; their MVP returned. A control group of 26 women with normal weight had 2 members with MVP. Incidentally, none of the women with MVP had chest pain or any other chest symptoms at any time.

Even low incidence groups, such as men in general and older men in particular, are found to have an MVP incidence of around 2%. The percentages quoted do not seem high, but when we apply them to the 230 million people in the U.S., we can conclude that between 5 and 10 million have MVP. All but a small fraction of these live a normal lifetime, unaware of the condition; any problems they have appear to be caused by associated or other diseases and not by the bulging of the mitral valve itself.

D. MVP and chest pain

Studies of various groups have demonstrated no connection between MVP and chest pain. The problem is much like that we saw for patient #5 in chapter I. Someone develops chest pain, frequently of the type we have called "neurocirculatory asthenia" (chapter IV). A number of examinations and tests are done and no physical cause for the pain is found. An echocardiogram shows MVP. The temptation to blame MVP for the pain is very great; tying the two together solves a number of problems for patient and doctor both.

In unusual situations MVP and cardiac pain can occur together, but there is no evidence of a cause and effect relationship. Both are the result of underlying ischemic heart disease. If ischemia happens to affect the papillary muscles (fig. 6, p. 51) one or more may weaken or even rupture. The attached valve will prolapse. This is not a common occurrence.

E. MVP and sudden death

Similarly, there is no good evidence that MVP causes sudden death. Again, we must make a very clear distinction between MVP—the bulging of the valve into the atrium—and the various situations in which it shows up. There are a few uncommon diseases in which MVP, sudden death, or both may occur. They are principally conditions in which there is abnormality and weakening of the connective tissue of the body. The mitral valve is mostly connective tissue. If this tissue weakens, the valve may bulge into the atrium; further weakening may allow the valve to tear or to become incompetent—that is, allow backflow of blood. Backward flow of blood may cause heart failure, lung congestion, and sometimes death. Chordae tendineae are also connective tissue; they may weaken and tear, causing similar problems. Sudden death sometimes occurs in these diseases even when there are no valve abnormalities.

Blood clots may form on valves in some situations. Parts of the clots may break off and go to one or more body organs, causing problems. Damaged valves are also susceptible to infection.

Echocardiography is done in many of the above situations. Some of the damaged valves prolapse, so it is not surprising that MVP is found in association with a wide variety of problems.

Even when valve disease is present, sudden death associated with MVP is rare. The authors of a recent paper on the subject (1983) found 39 cases reported in the entire literature to which they added 14 cases they had collected over 8 years. This is 53 total cases reported. Contrast this with 550,000 deaths yearly from ischemic heart disease. Even allowing for gross underreporting, it is evident that the incidence of sudden death associated with MVP of any kind is very low.

Nevertheless, the risk of serious problems and complications from diseases in which MVP is sometimes seen is real. MVP may be a major lead in the diagnosis of these diseases. For this reason MVP should be carefully evaluated by a competent physician whenever it is discovered; any problem found should be treated appropriately. It must still be emphasized that the evidence is that it is not the bulging of the valve into the atrium but the condition causing the bulge that is important.

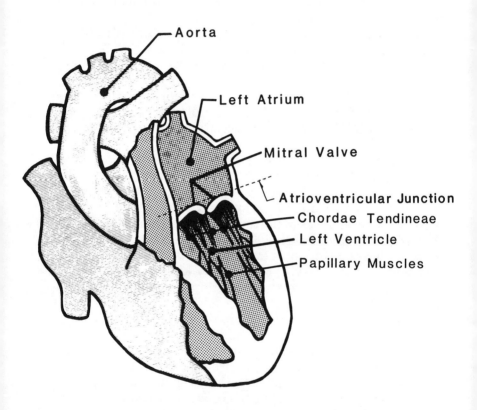

Aorta

Left Atrium

Mitral Valve

Atrioventricular Junction

Chordae Tendineae

Left Ventricle

Papillary Muscles

Mitral Valve

Fig. 8

74

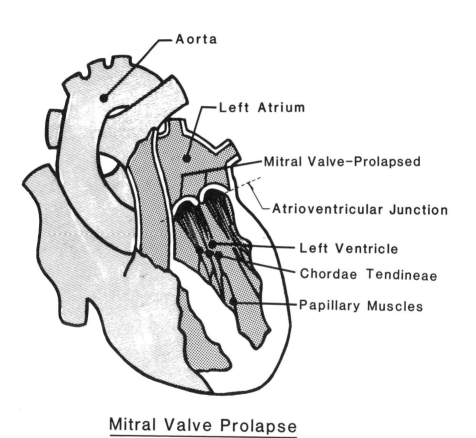

Aorta

Left Atrium

Mitral Valve–Prolapsed

Atrioventricular Junction

Left Ventricle

Chordae Tendineae

Papillary Muscles

Mitral Valve Prolapse

Fig. 9

75

Chapter Seven

TESTS FOR ISCHEMIC HEART DISEASE

A. Summary

Tests for ischemic heart disease fall into 3 groups: electrical, chemical, and imaging.

The heart produces an electric current which changes continuously through the cardiac cycle of contraction and relaxation. This current, measured in a number of different directions on the body, can be made to produce a graphic recording called the electrocardiogram (abbreviated ECG or EKG). The machine making the recording is called the electrocardiograph. Properly and cautiously interpreted the ECG is very useful but not foolproof. Normal ECGs can be recorded in the presence of heart disease and normal hearts can sometimes produce abnormal ECGs. In addition, there are a large number of ECG changes labelled "nonspecific" which can mean almost anything but usually mean nothing. The standard ECG is obtained in less than a minute at rest. Special recording monitors (Holter monitors) can be attached to patients to record their ECGs on tape over a period of 24 hours or more as they go about their normal activities. Another type of monitor shows the ECG continuously on a TV-like screen (oscilloscope).

The ECG usually but not always shows one of a number of characteristic patterns when cardiac ischemia is present. It was once thought that practically all episodes of cardiac ischemia were associated with pain. Monitors have demonstrated that many episodes of ischemia are painless.

The stress test is performed by subjecting the patient to progressively increasing work loads, usually by having him walk on a treadmill, and monitoring his ECG for ischemic changes during and after the test.

The ECG is also used to show changes in rate and rhythm. It is useful in separating harmless from dangerous variations (patient #5, chapter I).

Chemical tests measure the amounts of enzymes which escape from damaged heart cells into the blood. Enzymes are special compounds which speed up the chemical reactions necessary for cell life. Most enzymes are found in a number of different kinds of cells, so increased blood levels may not be helpful in deciding what organ is damaged. These increased levels are present only during the acute phase of the injury and last a few days at most. The enzyme called CK-MB (an abbreviation for creatine kinase, MB band), which is reasonably but not entirely specific for heart muscle, is very useful in evaluating cardiac injury.

Imaging procedures convert waves into pictures. The waves may be sound waves, light waves, radio waves, or the very short waves we call x-rays and gamma rays.

Echoes are reflections of sound waves. An echocardiogram is a pictorial representation of parts of the heart built up by timing echoes from these cardiac structures. Angiocardiograms are made by first injecting into the bloodstream substances which block x-rays; these are called contrast materials. X-rays of the heart and blood vessels are then made. The cavities of these structures are outlined on the films by the contrast material. Motion x-ray pictures made like this currently give the most accurate information about the heart and arteries. Pictures are also obtained from the gamma rays given off by radioactive elements which are injected and collect in parts of the heart.

Some atoms spinning in strong magnetic fields can be made to emit radio waves. Computers can transform these waves into pictures of the body structures containing the atoms. The process is called nuclear magnetic imaging. Most recently the insides of blood vessels are being looked at and photographed directly through long bundles of very thin flexible glass rods. This procedure is called angioscopy.

B. The electrocardiogram (ECG)

1. The ordinary (12 lead) ECG

The normal heartbeat starts with an electrical impulse in the right atrium at the SA node (fig. 7, p. 52). The contraction wave spreads through the atria, then the ventricles (systole). This is followed by a period of relaxation (diastole) during which the ventricles fill with blood and become electrically recharged (repolarized) for the next beat. Each phase, atrial contraction, ventricular contraction, and repolarization has its own characteristic electrical pattern; together they make up the pattern for one beat. The electrical impulse passes through the heart in 3 dimensions; we measure the electrical pattern on the chest wall from one point to another in a line. If we change the location of the contact points on the body, the pattern changes. It is customary to measure the electrical impulse in 12 leads; that is, in 12 different directions. The reason for this is that significant abnormalities may show up in only one or a few leads; the others may look normal. Special leads may sometimes pick up abnormalities not seen in the 12 standard leads.

It is not easy to understand an ECG without special training. Obvious changes like the pattern wandering on the paper and large vibrations up and down are meaningless; they are due to patient motion, loose leads, or electrical interference and have nothing to do with the heart. The changes we look for are much finer and very specific. Furthermore, there are many variations which are sometimes indications of disease and sometimes not.

One of the main uses of the ECG is to give corroborative evidence of the presence, location, and extent of ischemic heart disease. There are changes which are characteristic of this problem although they may occur in other conditions as well. If the changes go through a typical evolution over a period of time, the evidence for ischemic heart disease is strengthened. It is possible to have myocardial infarction without characteristic ECG changes and ECG changes without infarction.

The 12 lead ECG is useful in the diagnosis of rhythm disturbances. In people like patient #5 (chapter I) it helps to decide whether the extra beats are due to heart disease or not. It frequently establishes the cause of fast, slow, or irregular heartbeats.

2. Monitors

The 12 lead ECG takes less than a minute to record and tells us only about the heart's electrical activity at that time. If we need to follow cardiac behavior longer, we use monitors. These either show a continuous pattern on something like a TV screen (an oscilloscope) or record the pattern on tape for later study.

Oscilloscopes are used in hospitals and emergency ambulances to watch the heart action of patients with cardiac and other problems. Units are placed at the patient's bedside with a duplicate at the nurses' station. They usually have alarms that signal any important change or activity.

Tape monitors (Holter monitors) are ordinarily used for patients who are up and about in or out of the hospital. Some individuals have normal resting ECGs but there is a suspicion that their problems are due to a rhythm disturbance or cardiac ischemia which comes and goes. Portable monitors can record patterns for a day or more at a time; these can then be studied in detail later.

Monitors which report to the patient himself in "real time"—that is, at the instant something is happening—are just being released for use. They should provide much more information on patient status and treatment response, especially with such problems as silent ischemia (section 5 below). As they become more reliable and cheaper, their general use may allow us to identify more people at risk for complications earlier.

3. The stress test

Many times a patient will be suspected of having angina pectoris and will have a normal or relatively normal resting ECG. The stress test is performed by connecting the patient to a monitor and ECG machine and having him walk on a motor-driven treadmill. The speed and upward angle of the treadmill are gradually increased until: 1) the patient has chest pain, 2) monitor changes typical of ischemic heart disease appear, 3) the patient's heart speeds up to the target rate (usually about 85% of the maximum predicted for his age), or 4) the patient is forced by muscle pain or exhaustion to stop.

Either 1) or 2) is a positive test, 3) is a negative test, and 4) is considered incomplete or inconclusive. A negative test is good but far from certain evidence that the patient does not have classical angina pectoris (chapter II). The test is of little use in variant angina (chapter II).

The test is also of value in rhythm disturbances. A record that becomes normal or more nearly normal as the intensity of exercise increases is strong evidence that the dysrhythmia is not dangerous or a threat to life (patient #5, chapter I).

There is a small but definite risk in taking a stress test. The purpose of the test is to provoke the signs of ischemic heart disease if it is present. As with any such episode, whether spontaneous or provoked, there is danger of rhythm disturbances or even cardiac arrest. However, the test is done in the presence of a doctor with all the equipment at hand to take care of any problem that might arise. The test is stopped at the first sign that it is positive.

If the patient does not have ischemic heart disease, the risk does not arise. If he does, he presumably suffers many episodes of cardiac ischemia under more dangerous conditions than the stress test. The test is done to help determine whether the patient will need treatment for the rest of his life; the danger of neglecting the problem is much greater than the danger of the test. A consideration of the probable risk-benefit ratio (chapter V) usually decides that the test should be done if it is considered at all.

4. Other uses of the ECG

The ECG can provide evidence of congenital and acquired abnormalities of electrical pathways as well as abnormal thickening of or stress on cardiac muscle. Sometimes it is necessary to remove nodules of heart tissue which are the source of uncontrollable dangerous dysrhythmias; the ECG is useful in finding these nodules. The ECG is also an indispensable research tool.

5. Painless cardiac ischemia

Holter monitor tapes and stress test records often show unmistakable evidence of ischemia during periods when the patient is having no pain or any other symptom. Some reports show as many as 75% of ischemic episodes to be painless. Occasionally a patient will have a full-blown myocardial infarction without pain. Evidence of the past event appears on later ECGs or at surgery for subsequent problems. We do not know how many of the 15% of cardiac arrest victims with no history of chest pain (chapter II) have had episodes of painless ischemia before their arrests. This is a subject of much current research, but so far we have no certain explanation for the great variation in pain seen with cardiac ischemia. There is some evidence that painless episodes tend to be less severe than those with pain.

6. Dysrhythmia

The word dysrhythmia means disordered heart rhythm. The "normal" resting heart is supposed to beat regularly between 60 and 100 times a minute. Anything less than 60 is labelled bradycardia (slow heart); anything over 100 is tachycardia (fast heart). Resting bradycardia and tachycardia are not necessarily abnormal. A normal athlete can have a resting rate of 40 or less, and excitement can increase the rate of a normal heart to well above 100.

We discussed the dysrhythmias associated with cardiac arrest in chapter II. People with ischemic heart disease are at increased risk for the development of these as well as other rhythm disturbances. In chapter VIII we will talk about medications used to help prevent such problems. On the other hand, many dysrhythmias are harmless (patient #5, chapter I).

While we can usually tell that some abnormality of rhythm is present just by listening, it is frequently impossible to determine the exact nature of the problem and the best treatment without an ECG.

C. Chemical tests

Every cell in the body (chapter III) is a factory in which many different chemical reactions go on. The reactions are necessary for the cell to live and function. Enzymes are catalysts which help these reactions take place. Many specific enzymes are found in a large variety of different cell types, some occur in only a few types of cells, and occasionally one appears to be specific for a single type of cell, or nearly so.

Normally the levels of these intracellular enzymes circulating in blood are very low. When cells are damaged, as for instance by insufficient oxygen, they may leak some of these enzymes into the blood stream. An increased level of enzyme in the blood is an indication of cell damage.

The enzyme labelled CK-MB is the one currently most useful for indicating cardiac injury. For a while it was thought that increased levels came only from damaged heart muscle; now it is realized that there are other possible sources. For example, CK-MB may be elevated in marathon runners or in patients with skeletal muscle injury by electricity.

Other enzymes are released by damaged heart tissue, but they can come from other types of injured cells as well. Even so, their blood levels may be useful in following the course of cardiac damage.

D. Imaging procedures

An imaging procedure gives a picture or at least some type of graphic representation of the heart, coronary arteries, aorta, pulmonary arteries, or parts of these structures. In many, the area under investigation can be watched directly on a screen while the picture is being made. The procedures in general use are: 1) ordinary x-rays, 2) studies with radioactive elements, 3) ultrasonography, 4) angiography, 5) nuclear magnetic imaging, 6) angioscopy.

1. Chest x-ray

Ordinary x-rays may be very useful in the evaluation of pain coming from other chest structures, but they usually do not help much with the cardiac variety. They can tell us if the heart is enlarged or abnormal in shape, or if there is a large amount of fluid in or around the lungs. They may make us suspicious of an aortic aneurysm (chapter II). Rarely do they tell us anything about ischemic heart disease directly.

2. Radioactive elements (radionuclides)

Radioactive elements break down to give off rays like x-rays except that they are even more penetrating. Like x-rays they make a picture (after suitable processing) when they strike photographic film. The 2 elements in common use are technetium 99 and thallium 201. They are used to outline areas of injured heart muscle because they collect preferentially in the damaged or normal muscle.

If the history, physical examination, ECG, and chemical tests do not give sufficient information about the existence or extent of cardiac damage, radionuclide studies are sometimes done next. They can be used during a stress test to show the presence of decreased flow to a part of the heart. The radiation dose and chemical toxicity of these agents are negligible; they require only an injection into an arm vein before the pictures are taken, so they are nearly free of risk.

3. Ultrasonography, echocardiography

Ultrasonography is the use of ultrasound waves to make pictures. Echocardiography is the name of this process applied to the heart. Ultrasound waves are sound waves of much higher pitch than can be heard by the human ear. They are reflected from boundaries such as boundaries between liquids and solids and boundaries between solids and solids. In echocardiographic studies these waves are produced in short bursts lasting about a millionth of a second; the rate is about a thousand bursts per second. The speed of the waves in the human body is known very accurately; the turnaround time of the sound pulse can also be measured accurately. The distances from boundaries to the instrument and the distances between boundaries are calculated by the computer in the instrument, which then uses the numbers to build a picture.

The heart can be thought of as a series of boundaries: the boundary between the outer heart wall and lung, the boundaries between the inner heart walls and blood, the boundaries between valve leaflets and blood on both sides of the leaflets, and so on. The machine builds a graphic representation of the heart from the information it obtains, but the picture looks nothing like a heart and must be interpreted by experts. It is useful in evaluating such things as abnormal heart wall thickness and motion as well as variations in valve thickness and mobility. Echocardiography is the method used to detect mitral valve prolapse (chapter VI). Since it employs only sound waves there are no known risks attending its use.

4. Contrast angiography

As far as x-rays are concerned, blood, arterial wall, and cardiac tissue all have about the same density. This makes plain x-rays almost useless for visualizing details of heart and coronary artery internal structure. If, however, material that blocks x-rays is dissolved in the blood, these internal structures can be outlined. Such materials are called contrast media; they usually contain iodine compounds, since iodine effectively blocks x-rays.

For best definition the contrast medium must be placed directly into the heart chambers or coronary arteries. This requires passing a thin tube (catheter) into an arm or leg artery, into the aorta, then into a coronary artery at the aortic valve (fig. 4, p. 49) or through the aortic valve into the left ventricle (fig. 3, p. 48).

The procedure is more complex and expensive than any we have described so far. There is a small risk of damage to an artery from catheter insertion and a similar small risk of serious rhythm disturbances from contrast material. Allergic reactions to contrast media also occur. On the other hand, contrast studies provide information that cannot be obtained in any other way. They are especially important if any type of surgical procedure is being considered. Weak areas in the left ventricular wall can be mapped and proper corrective procedures planned. Valve and other problems can be precisely defined and the best treatment chosen. The location, number, and extent of atherosclerotic coronary deposits can be visualized to allow the choice of proper therapy. Congenital abnormalities can also be seen, if they are present.

Coronary arteriography has demonstrated that 85% to 90% of myocardial infarctions are caused by blood clots developing on atherosclerotic plaques. It has also been demonstrated that if treatment is started early (within a few hours of the onset of pain) the clot can frequently be dissolved and permanent heart damage minimized or even eliminated. As of now, coronary angiography is the gold standard of all our tests.

Digital subtraction angiography is related to contrast angiography but is not quite the same. First an x-ray of the chest is taken and stored in the computer. Contrast medium is then injected but this time into an arm vein; catheters in arteries are not used. X-rays are made as contrast medium spreads through the heart and blood vessels of the chest. The computer extracts the picture of the chest without contrast medium, so that only the blood vessel pictures remain.

This procedure is at first glance very attractive, since it involves only an intravenous injection and x-rays, and eliminates the elaborate and expensive setup needed to put catheters into arteries safely. However, it does not give as much clarity and definition as standard contrast angiography. Since these procedures are in most cases done to decide whether a patient has significant disease and whether and what kind of surgery is indicated, the best pictures and the most information obtainable are needed. In addition, the injection of the required large volumes of contrast material needed for subtraction angiography can lead to complications in some cases. For these reasons digital subtraction studies are not much used for coronary visualization.

5. Nuclear magnetic imaging

This procedure is just beginning to be used in medicine in general. Its use in heart problems is still largely experimental.

When strong magnetic fields are applied to atoms of some elements, those atoms develop characteristic spin patterns. Spinning atoms broadcast radio waves. These waves vary with the atom and its chemical environment; a computer converts them into a picture of the body area they are coming from. Since damaged heart muscle differs chemically from normal muscle, pictures of hearts with myocardial infarcts can be generated from living persons. So far the images cannot show enough fine detail to give useful information about coronary arteries.

The method uses only magnets and radio waves so it poses no known health hazard. It cannot be used by patients with pacemakers (chapter VIII) or metal implants. Also, the equipment installations are very expensive, costing millions of dollars. In spite of these drawbacks, the procedure shows very great promise and is likely to become one of our diagnostic mainstays in the near future.

6. Angioscopy

This is even newer than magnetic imaging. Long flexible bundles of very thin glass rods are used to look inside blood vessels in living humans. Similar instruments have been used for some time in the examination of the gastrointestinal and respiratory tracts. The inside of the pulmonary artery has been visualized by passing such a bundle into a large vein in the neck, through the right atrium and ventricle, into the artery. The insides of human coronary arteries have been examined but so far only by introducing the bundle directly into the artery with the heart exposed at surgery.

New as the method is, it has already provided one useful observation. Cases of unstable angina (chapter II) have been demonstrated by direct vision to be due to the formation and breaking up of clots on atherosclerotic plaques. The future of angioscopy will depend on how far refinements in instrumentation can be carried.

Chapter Eight

TREATMENT

A. Summary

This chapter will discuss the treatment of the complications of coronary atherosclerosis: angina pectoris, myocardial infarction, and cardiac arrest. So far as the treatment of uncomplicated atherosclerosis itself is concerned, there are surgical procedures for removing or flattening atherosclerotic plaques; we are not sure that any of our medical methods are effective for this purpose. Even with effective methods it would be hard to find the right people to treat, since uncomplicated atherosclerosis has no signs or symptoms (chapter V). Prevention of atherosclerosis will be discussed in chapter IX.

Treatment may be medical, surgical, or both. Medical treatment is the use of drugs and lifestyle changes to accomplish one or more of the following: increase cardiac blood flow, decrease cardiac work, decrease dysrhythmias, prevent blood clot formation in the coronary arteries, or dissolve any clots that form. Medicines used are nitro compounds, beta adrenergic blocking agents, calcium channel blockers, special drugs for dysrhythmias, medicines to prevent clot formation, and medicines to dissolve clots.

Surgical procedures are used to improve blood supply

to part of the heart, implant devices to treat dysrhythmias, remove tissue which may be a source of dysrhythmias, repair weak spots or tears in heart tissue, or implant devices or donor hearts to assist or replace the heart. With so many different modalities available, treatment must obviously be carefully matched to the needs of the individual patient.

B. Angina pectoris

1. Medical treatment

The pain, rhythm disturbances, and cardiac arrest associated with angina are the result of inadequate blood supply to part of the heart. One way to handle the problem is to decrease activity, excitement, and so on, to keep cardiac work load down. Most people find the practicality of this approach limited. However, lifestyle changes to cut down stress are highly desirable for angina patients.

Medications are used in angina for the following purposes: 1) to dilate coronary arteries and allow more blood to flow through them, 2) to decrease incoming blood load on the heart, 3) to decrease the oxygen consumption of the heart, 4) to decrease the irritability of the heart and make dangerous dysrhythmias less likely, 5) to decrease clot formation, 6) to dissolve clots. Medicines used are: 1) nitro compounds, 2) beta adrenergic blocking agents, 3) calcium channel blockers, 4) special antidysrhythmic agents, 5) drugs which interfere with the clotting process at various points.

1.a. Nitro compounds

These medications act by dilating the blood vessels of the body to decrease the load on the heart and by dilating coronary arteries to allow more blood to get to ischemic heart tissues; some researchers doubt that this second mechanism is of much importance. Nitroglycerin is the most commonly used medicine in this group. Placed under the tongue it usually relieves the pain of angina in 2 or 3 minutes. Cardiac pain not relieved by nitroglycerin suggests that either the nitroglycerin is too old or that the patient may be having a myocardial infarction rather than just an anginal attack.

Nitroglycerin is effective but short acting. It is sometimes incorporated into pastes or other carriers for application to the skin to prolong its activity. There is some evidence that skin application is less and less effective with repeated use. Longer activity can also be obtained by using other nitro compounds such as isosorbide dinitrate taken by mouth.

1.b. Beta adrenergic blocking agents

Adrenergic compounds are substances like adrenaline manufactured by the body and by chemists. Depending on which ones we are talking about, they increase the rate and strength of heartbeats, constrict the blood vessels of the body, and open the small air passages of the lungs, among their other effects. They are very important in the body's "fight or flight" response to danger, real or imagined. Unfortunately, they also increase the heart's oxygen requirement and increase its irritability, making it more sensitive to dangerous dysrhythmias. Large amounts of adrenergic agents may be produced by the body as a result of physical or emotional stress.

This tendency to dysrhythmias becomes worse in ischemic heart disease, where decreased oxygen supply has already made cardiac tissue irritable. To counteract these cardiac effects (the beta effects), beta blocking agents have been developed. They have become very important in the treatment of angina and myocardial infarction, and are almost routinely prescribed if the patient has no contraindications. They must be used only in carefully evaluated patients, as they may aggravate such problems as asthma, congestive heart failure, and slow or blocked beats.

1.c. Calcium channel blockers

Calcium is a chemical element which is necessary for the contraction of all muscle, including heart muscle and the muscle cells of arterial walls. Calcium is also important in the function of parts of the conduction system of the heart. Calcium channel blockers partially block the entrance of calcium into cells, decreasing the contractility of some muscle and the conductivity of some cardiac tissue. Not all of these agents affect all cells equally. There are 3 blockers in current use in the U.S. One affects chiefly cardiac muscle and connective tissue, the second works mainly on smooth muscle of arterial walls, and the third combines some of the characteristics of the first two. The choice of which if any of these to use obviously depends on the problems the patient is having.

1.d. Antidysrhythmic agents

There is a group of drugs which are primarily anti-dysrhythmic agents. Patients in the acute phase of a myocardial infarction and patients who have been resuscitated from a cardiac arrest are especially likely to develop (or redevelop) dysrhythmias. Antidysrhythmic agents are used almost routinely for prevention and treatment in such circumstances. Other ischemic heart disease patients continue to have rhythm problems in spite of apparently adequate treatment; antidysrhythmics are used in these as well.

1.e. Drugs to control clot formation and dissolve clots

Blood clotting is a complex process which involves special cell products called platelets plus a number of chemicals manufactured by the body. Clots are necessary to prevent blood loss from injury. However, clots blocking intact blood vessels can cause serious damage or death.

Platelets are tiny fragments, smaller than red blood cells, which are released by special cells in the bone marrow. They can start a clot by sticking to a damaged area of inner blood vessel wall. More platelets join the first ones, forming a clump. Clumping initiates a series of chemical reactions resulting in a clot. We attempt to interfere with this process at 3 levels: 1) medicines such as aspirin make platelets less sticky and less likely to stick to vessel walls and each other; 2) medicines like heparin and Coumadin interfere with the clotting reaction series by a variety of mechanisms; 3) medicines like streptokinase (patient #2, chapter I) and tissue plasminogen activator (abbreviated TPA) activate the body's mechanism for dissolving clots.

The chief problem seen with these medicines, as might be expected, is excessive bleeding. With careful control this is rarely a major problem, but patients and physicians must be alert for the possibility.

1.f. Conclusion

The choice of which type of medicine to use first, second, and third, which of the medicines in each class to use, and which if any classes to combine can only be made by a competent physician after careful evaluation of the individual patient. Response to these drugs varies so much from patient to patient that it is frequently necessary to try many regimens to find the best one.

Many patients do very well on medical treatment. Their pain is controlled and some regression of their atherosclerosis appears to take place. This is especially true if known risk factors (chapter IX) are brought under control. Sometimes, however, the disease progresses or makes itself known at such a late stage that medical control alone is unlikely. In such cases surgery should be considered.

2. Surgery

Surgical procedures for ischemic heart disease fall into several classes: 1) procedures to improve blood supply to part of the heart, 2) procedures to implant devices to treat dysrhythmias that cannot successfully be treated with drugs, 3) procedures to repair mechanically weak or torn areas of the heart, 4) procedures to remove tissue which is a source of dysrhythmias, 5) procedures to implant devices or donor hearts to assist or replace the heart.

2.a. Procedures to improve blood supply

2.a.1). Coronary bypass

In this procedure blood vessels from some other part of the body are used to carry blood around one or more blocked or partly blocked sections of coronary artery. The vessels used are usually the saphenous vein from the leg or the internal mammary artery from the chest wall near the breastbone. Removal of these vessels causes no blood supply problem in the leg or chest. One end of the vessel is sewn into the aorta and the other into a coronary branch on the other side of the block. The requirements are that the disease be sufficiently localized so that the important blocks can be bypassed and that the coronary bed on the other side of the blocks be open enough to make the procedure worthwhile. These conditions are verified by coronary angiography (chapter VII) before surgery. Sometimes the disease is so widespread that the operation is unlikely to be helpful.

The consensus now is that this is an excellent procedure when indicated. Patient #1 (chapter I) had a very good result. As with anything else in medicine, there can be complications and failures. In the best hands—meaning experienced, competent surgeons and institutions that do many procedures— operative mortality is now around 1% and bad results (more pain after surgery) around 5%. About 50% of the patients overall become pain free and most of the rest show improvement. Much depends on the condition of the patient and his heart. Statistics such as those above are overall; they include patients with advanced scarring as well as patients in good condition with localized blocks and no scarring. The patient with minimal disease is more likely to have an excellent result, but many people with advanced atherosclerosis have been helped greatly as well.

2.a.2). Balloon angioplasty

This procedure is new. It was developed in Switzerland around 1977 and has been widely used in this country for only the past 3 or 4 years. The official name is a jaw-breaker: percutaneous transluminal coronary angioplasty, abbreviated PTCA.

Coronary angiography (chapter VII) is first performed to locate the obstructions that are to be dilated. Not all patients or obstructions are suitable candidates for PTCA. However, equipment is improving so rapidly and use of the procedure is being extended so much that anything written now about indications or limitations will be out of date before it is printed.

A deflated balloon attached to a long tube is passed over a guide into an artery (usually in the groin), then into the aorta, then into a coronary artery. Small squirts of contrast material and x-ray imaging on a TV screen allow the balloon to be introduced under direct visual control. The balloon is positioned in the center of the obstructed segment of coronary artery and inflated. This squeezes the cholesterol and other material in the plaque out into the wall of the artery, widening the channel.

The procedure is done with the patient awake. He usually goes home the next day or the day after. About one time in 50 the artery splits and blood seeps into the wall; the procedure is done with a surgical team standing by so the artery can be bypassed immediately if necessary. The patient may develop dysrhythmias during the dilatation: these are usually easily controlled. As with bypass surgery, there may be other complications. As many as 25% may have to have the procedure repeated in 6 to 8 months. With repeats, the overall success rate (again in experienced hands) is now about 80%. This is the procedure which was done on patient #2 (chapter

I). So far, approximately 21 months after the operation, his results are excellent.

2.a.3). Endarterectomy

Endarterectomy involves the shelling out of the inner layer of the artery with its plaques. A new inner lining then grows back, resurfacing the arterial channel. This is still sometimes done, but usually in conjunction with bypass procedures.

2.a.4). Laser surgery; electric knives

A laser is a concentrated thin beam of light. It can be used to deliver energy to tiny areas for precise cutting. The energy can be made so intense that it will turn to gas anything in the very small area the beam touches without damaging nearby structures.

Lasers have been used in medicine for several years. Very recent applications have been to burn holes in obstructions inside arteries and to partially remove atherosclerotic plaques by vaporizing plaque material. This work is still in its early experimental stages; no one knows when or whether the method will come into general use. Even more recently small electric knives on the end of long flexible rods have been used experimentally to shave down plaques.

2.b. Dysrhythmia treatment

2.b.1). Pacemakers

A pacemaker is a device that delivers tiny electric shocks to the heart to serve as artificial heartbeat starters. With the internal pacemaker the shocks are delivered through a wire or wires implanted directly into the heart.

The SA node (fig. 7, p. 52) is the normal source of the impulse that initiates each heartbeat. Sometimes the node or some part of the heart's conduction system is damaged. This may result in partial or complete interruption of the formation of impulses for contractions or their travel through the heart. Such interruptions may be temporary, intermittent, or permanent. Some other part of the heart may take over the pacemaker job, but the substitute is rarely reliable. Transient problems may be treated with medicines. When these are not successful an artificial internal pacemaker, usually fixed so that it generates an electrical impulse or impulses when the heart misses, is installed. In an emergency the pacer wire is passed through the skin into a central vein and into the heart. The pulse generator, powered by a small battery, is taped to the chest.

If the situation straightens itself out the temporary pacer can be removed. If the deficit appears to be irreversible, the temporary pacer must be replaced by a permanent one. The pulse generator is implanted under the skin and the pacer wire is led first under the skin, then into the chest to the heart.

External pacemakers, in which the voltage is applied to the intact skin through 2 electrodes placed so that the heart is between them, are sometimes used in acute emergencies. If pacing needs to be continued for any length of time they are replaced by the temporary or permanent internal variety.

2.b.2). Intractable dysrhythmias
A few patients have dangerous dysrhythmias which cannot be controlled by medicines. Sometimes there is a small area of the heart which is the source of the abnormal electrical impulses. These areas can often be removed surgically with good results.

2.c. Weak spots; ventricular aneurysms
Part of the wall of a ventricle (almost always the left) may be damaged and weakened sufficiently so that instead of contracting with the rest of the ventricle during systole it bulges out. Some of the blood that should be going to the aorta is pumped into the bulge with each beat. The weakness may be progressive and the bulge (called an aneurysm) may rupture; such a rupture may be immediately fatal.

Aneurysms can be repaired surgically. The immediate results are usually good but clots forming inside the ventricle at the repair site can be a problem.

√ 2.d. Ventricular assist and replacement
The ventricles (fig. 5, p. 50) do about 95% of the work in pumping blood, with the left doing 4 or 5 times as much as the right, normally. The left ventricle is the one most commonly damaged by ischemic heart disease; it is the one that usually fails first from such damage. Some devices are designed to assist the left ventricle, others to assist or replace the whole heart.

2.d.1). Intraaortic balloon pump

This device consists of a balloon on the end of a tube. The balloon is deflated and threaded through the femoral artery (the large artery in the groin, chapter III) into the aorta. The balloon is connected to a gas supply and pump which inflate it during diastole and deflate it during systole with each heartbeat. This has the effect of partly emptying the aorta into the body during diastole and allowing it to fill against a very low pressure during systole. The overall effect is to decrease the work load on the heart. The balloon is a temporary expedient. It is used to gain time until there is improvement in heart action or until some definitive procedure can be performed.

✕ 2.d.2). Artificial hearts

So far these are experimental. They have kept humans alive for over a year, although with multiple complications. The most successful model to date must be powered by a bulky outside pump. Many problems will have to be solved before a totally implantable unit can be made to work. Nevertheless, because of the difficulties with large scale use of heart transplants, development of such a unit for patients whose hearts are no longer salvageable is very much to be hoped for.

✕ 2.d.3). Heart transplants

These are being done at a number of places in the U.S. The results continue to improve. The longest that a transplant patient has lived so far is 13 years after the operation. More than 40% of the most recent group from a large center have lived over 5 years. Since these patients had a life expectancy measured in weeks or less before surgery, the numbers are impressive. The problems remain scarcity of suitable donors, difficulties in tissue matching, and the tremendous investment in time, money, and other resources required for each patient.

Transplants of hearts from animals have so far not been successful; they may be a possibility for the future.

C. Myocardial infarction (MI)

We have defined myocardial infarction (abbreviated MI) as irreversible damage to heart tissue (meaning cell death and eventual replacement by scar tissue) caused by inadequate blood supply. Although severe continued coronary artery spasm may at times be responsible, in the great majority of cases the cause is a blood clot forming on an atherosclerotic plaque.

The introduction of effective clot dissolving agents has left us with a problem in definition. In the past, when a patient came in with a typical pattern of pain, unresponsiveness to medication, and (usually) electrocardiographic changes, we could be reasonably sure that that individual would develop some permanent heart damage no matter what we did. With the use of clot dissolvers it appears that some of these people escape with no evidence of heart damage that we can find. Technically, they have not had MIs. Nevertheless, we continue to classify and treat them as such for the first 24 to 48 hours since for that period they may still be subject to the same risks as with the full-blown MI.

An MI is a true emergency and must be treated immediately. Patient #2 (chapter I) was started on standard treatment: oxygen, nitrates, beta blockers, and antidysrhythmics. All these are given to minimize pain and prevent complications as far as possible. While they may help to decrease tissue destruction, they do nothing about the clot and infarction process itself. As of this writing, streptokinase is the only clot dissolving agent available for general use. Streptokinase was given to patient #2. His clot dissolved and, so far as we can tell, he recovered with no permament heart damage.

Tissue plasminogen activator (TPA), a substance which occurs naturally in the body and, like streptokinase, activates the body's own clot dissolving mechanism, appears to be safer and more effective than streptokinase. Hopefully by the time this reaches print TPA will be available for general use. Agents that appear to be even better are under development.

The chief problem is time. Salvage of heart muscle drops off rapidly; after 4 hours these medicines do not seem to help much. Ideally they should be given much sooner if possible. There is no way to be sure, but part of the very good result that patient #2 had was probably because he was given streptokinase within an hour after the onset of his pain.

All of the medicines and surgical procedures described under treatment for angina (section B of this chapter) can be and are used as needed in the patient recovering from an MI. In particular, the use of beta blocking agents has been shown to decrease the incidence of cardiac arrest in this group. Carefully supervised exercise programs are also helpful at times. As with patient #2, most patients recovering from an MI have coronary angiography done to aid in the choice of proper treatment, whether medical, surgical, or both. Timing of angiography must be individualized.

D. Cardiac arrest
This is the most dreaded complication of ischemic heart disease. The heart stops beating effectively; no blood gets to the body and brain. Unless basic cardiopulmonary resuscitation (CPR) is started in 4 minutes and advanced cardiac life support is started within 8 minutes of the arrest, the patient's chances of surviving are small. These 4 and 8 minute limits do not apply to some patients and some problems. Childhood arrest, electrical injuries, and cold water drowning are examples of situations in which recovery has occurred after much longer times. The 4 and 8 minute limits do unfortunately apply to the great majority of ischemic heart disease patients.

Basic CPR consists of rhythmic chest compression to pump blood and mouth-to-mouth respiration to get oxygen into the patient's lungs. The American Heart Association gives courses in CPR nationwide; everyone over the age of 8 should have this training.

Advanced cardiac life support (ACLS) involves the use of intravenous drugs, electrical defibrillation, and complicated airway techniques. The necessary medicines and equipment are almost never available outside of ambulances and hospitals, so there is not much point in teaching the skills needed to anyone except medical personnel. The American Heart Association has special ACLS courses for this purpose.

Most of the time the dysrhythmia responsible for sudden cardiac arrest is ventricular fibrillation (chapter II). This can occur in hearts with relatively little coronary artery disease. About 85% of people who have cardiac arrests have had chest pain at some previous time. Adequate, timely medical care would cut down the number of arrests in this group.

When we consider the communication and transportation difficulties in most of our major cities, let alone our rural areas, a major increase in the number of arrest victims getting ACLS in 8 minutes will be hard to achieve. Another approach is to try to extend the 8 minute limit. This has been done experimentally. Cells do not die in 8 minutes; lack of oxygen sets in motion processes which cause further break-down leading to cell death later. Much current research is being done on ways to stop and reverse these secondary changes.

The great majority of patients who arrest do so because of coronary atherosclerosis, although many do not appear to have clots when their hearts are examined. This observation may be misleading, since clots can form, cause arrest, and dissolve rapidly.

As with angina and MI patients, the post-arrest victim should have a complete workup to decide on the best continuing treatment. About 25% of arrest victims have another arrest within a year. The treatment methods described under Angina (section B, this chapter) are used in patients recovering from cardiac arrest as well.

Chapter Nine

PREVENTION

A. Summary

✗ People have large inborn differences in the way their bodies handle cholesterol. In addition, there are external risk factors that influence how much coronary atherosclerosis develops and how much trouble it causes. A few lucky individuals can do as they like about these risk factors and have no apparent problems; for most of us risk factor control makes a big difference.

Smoking, high blood pressure, diabetes, and high blood cholesterol all lead to increased atherosclerosis. Everyone agrees that these cause serious problems. Not everyone agrees on their relative importance or on the safety and desirability of some of the measures used to control them. There is even more disagreement on the importance of obesity, lack of exercise, and the so-called type A or "coronary" personality.

There has been a 39% drop in death rate from ischemic heart disease and a correspondingly steep drop in deaths from stroke in the U.S. in the past 20 years. This means a saving of about 400,000 lives each year. During this period people have been smoking less, eating less cholesterol and animal fat, and exercising more. Some of the drop in death rate has been due to improved medical care, but the most likely causes for the major part of the drop are the changes in smoking, diet, and exercise.

The safety of some of these health habits has been questioned. However, except for lung cancer and chronic lung disease, there has been no appreciable increase in deaths from any cause in this same 20 year period. The saving in lives is real; we appear to be on the right track.

B. Introduction

Obviously the best way to prevent strokes, angina, myocardial infarction, and cardiac arrest is to prevent atherosclerosis in the first place. Prevention measures are hard to evaluate. Atherosclerotic plaques usually develop slowly and erratically over a period of years. For most of this time they show no sign of their presence. Tracking the progress of plaques in people during this silent period is not easy. The best method we have for detecting early lesions, coronary angiography (chapter VII), is not suited to mass screening. Most adults in the U.S. have some coronary atherosclerosis; it might be difficult, even if we could find the affected individuals, to tell which ones are going to get worse and develop complications.

No animal develops atherosclerosis in the same way a human does. Many animals can be made to develop the disease by special feeding; some treatment and prevention measures can be evaluated in these. How much of the animal research is applicable to humans is in many cases hard to decide.

Atherosclerosis is not restricted to the coronary arteries. We have already talked about its importance in causing aortic aneurysms and blocks in the lower aorta and leg arteries (chapter II). It also occurs in the arteries supplying the brain; obstruction of those by atherosclerosis and clots is the main cause of strokes. Strokes are the third leading cause of death in the U.S. after ischemic heart disease and cancer.

People are born with large variations in their ability to handle cholesterol without deposit formation. However, there are a number of external risk factors which profoundly affect the amount, severity, and complications of atherosclerosis that actually develop.

Many studies on the prevention of atherosclerosis have been done. They provide textbook examples of all the problems described in the chapter on Statistics and Proof (chapter V) and many more besides. What follows in this chapter is an outline of the opinions of many people who are doing active research in the field. However, there will be some disagreement with almost any statement we make.

In spite of the difficulties, long term prospective studies are beginning to give us definite answers. Smoking, high blood pressure, diabetes, and blood cholesterol elevation accelerate the progress and severity of atherosclerosis. Closely associated with cholesterol level is the way cholesterol is distributed among its blood carriers. Diet is a major determinant of both level and distribution. Lack of exercise, obesity, and type A or "coronary" personality are considered by some but not all researchers to be important. Each of these will be discussed in more detail.

C. Smoking

Cigarette smoking has been established beyond doubt as something which increases the incidence of atherosclerosis and its complications. The connection between cigarettes and lung disease is well known and very strong. While the odds are not quite so bad with atherosclerosis, the smoker can expect to increase greatly his chances of problems with ischemic heart disease if he continues the habit. The effect is cumulative; every cigarette smoked in a lifetime adds to the risk. Conversely, anyone who quits or cuts down at any time is better off than anyone who does not. It is not easy to stop smoking, but it is worth the effort.

D. High blood pressure

High blood pressure (hypertension) is a well established risk factor for atherosclerosis and ischemic heart disease. Unfortunately, disappointingly small benefits have been shown so far from treatment of groups of people with blood pressure medications. The reasons are not hard to find. While people may be aware of sudden large increases in blood pressure, sustained high blood pressure usually causes no symptoms until disaster strikes. Treatment is a classic example of trying to get people to take medicine for years and years when they cannot tell that it is doing them a particle of good (chapter V). As a result, medications are often taken irregularly if at all. Secondly, many doctors do not view hypertension as a serious problem unless it is severe. They may be less than enthusiastic about attempts at adequate control. Finally, 1 or 2 blood pressure medicines appear to create problems with blood cholesterol. No one knows how important this is, but it is a source of concern.

We do have safe and effective blood pressure medicines. Proper control for large numbers of people with hypertension would make a sizable additional dent in our ischemic heart disease mortality rate (see section J below).

Blood pressure is measured in millimeters of mercury and is given as 2 numbers, the systolic and diastolic pressure. Systolic pressure is the highest pressure developed in large arteries at the peak of cardiac contraction (systole). Diastolic pressure is the pressure in the arteries when the heart is relaxed (diastole). The pressures vary some from artery to artery. By long standing custom any pressure over 140 systolic or 90 diastolic measured by standard blood pressure cuff in the large artery in the upper arm is considered to be hypertension.

For many years emphasis was placed on diastolic pressure. It has been found, however, that increased systolic pressure is also associated with increased ischemic heart disease. Both systolic and diastolic pressure are important. Also, the sharp dividing line at 140 for systolic pressure appears to be misleading; there is a slight increase in risk at systolic levels above 105. We now have many effective and safe medications for the treatment of hypertension. The uncertainties concern the level at which we should start treatment and the blood pressure we should try to attain.

Ease of blood pressure control varies from person to person, so decisions must be individualized. Many doctors still use the 140 dividing line; others do not. The presence of other risk factors has some bearing on this. Obesity and emotional stress may be precipitating or aggravating factors for increased blood pressure. They should be controlled as much as possible in hypertensive people.

E. Diabetes

Diabetes is a disorder in which the patient is unable to burn sugar properly because of a relative or absolute lack of insulin. It is characterized by a high blood sugar which in turn allows some sugar to spill into the urine.

Diabetes is accompanied by increased atherosclerosis and by an increased risk of ischemic heart disease. It is generally but not universally accepted that reasonable control of blood sugar by weight reduction, diet, medicines by mouth, and/or insulin will decrease the amount of atherosclerosis.

It is possible to go overboard with this approach. High blood sugar is bad in the long run, but attempts at too rigorous control can lead to episodes of low blood sugar which present an immediate danger. Low blood sugar can cause abnormal behavior, coma which may become irreversible, or death. There is a widespread misconception that oral drugs for diabetes cannot cause dangerously low blood sugar. They can, especially if taken along with certain other medications.

F. Cholesterol

Cholesterol is a compound of the class called steroids. Steroids are a very large group of chemicals characterized by a special 4 ring arrangement of carbon atoms. Other steroids in the body are sex hormones like testosterone and adrenal hormones like hydrocortisone. Cholesterol and related materials are the main substances found in atherosclerotic plaques. Cholesterol is also a necessary constituent of body cells. We absorb it from foods of animal origin (plants do not have any) and our bodies manufacture it.

Increased blood cholesterol level is associated with an increased risk of ischemic heart disease. This has long been recognized for levels over 260 milligrams per 100 cc of blood, present in about 10% of Americans over the age of 40. Levels below this were considered normal because they were found in the majority of the population.

It now appears that our "normals" are really high and are caused mainly by a high intake of fat, especially animal fat. The risk of ischemic heart disease increases as the cholesterol level rises above 180 milligrams per 100 cc; the higher the level, the higher the risk. The current recommendation from the National Institute of Health is that people under 30 with levels above 200, under 40 with levels above 220, and over 40 with levels over 240 take steps to bring their levels down to these values or lower.

Control consists essentially of decreasing fat, especially animal fat, in the diet and taking medication if necessary. The situation is complicated by the fact that there is still much we do not know about the way the body handles cholesterol. Almost no cholesterol can dissolve in water or blood directly. Cholesterol is picked up and carried around in blood by special proteins; the combination of protein with cholesterol and other fats is called a lipoprotein. There are several kinds of lipoprotein in blood, but the two that concern us most are low density lipoprotein (LDL) and high density lipoprotein (HDL). Most cholesterol is carried as LDL; when total cholesterol rises the increase is almost always in this fraction. Body cells normally have receptors for LDL; they attach to the LDL, then the cell internalizes the cholesterol and uses it. If the receptors are decreased in number, absent, or not working right, blood LDL level rises and cholesterol deposits in artery walls, forming plaques.

In contrast to LDL, HDL seems to take cholesterol out of the tissues and so decrease plaque formation. There is much less HDL than LDL in blood and much less variation in blood level; nevertheless, both the amount of HDL and the ratio of HDL to LDL appear to be important determinants of plaque formation. Anything that raises HDL or lowers LDL is beneficial; anything that lowers HDL or raises LDL is harmful. To make matters more difficult, HDL can be split into fractions; only one of these appears to be effective in removing cholesterol from tissues.

In addition to other factors, blood cholesterol level depends on the amount of fat we eat, the kind of fat we eat, and how much cholesterol we eat. The less cholesterol we eat the less we have in our blood. Cholesterol is strictly an animal product. Vegetables contain none.

The effect of fat is more complicated. Fatty acids are the major parts of fat molecules; they come in different varieties. Saturated fatty acids contain no double bonds (can add no hydrogen); unsaturated fatty acids contain one double bond (can add 2 hydrogen atoms); polyunsaturated fatty acids contain 2 or more double bonds (can add 4 or more hydrogen atoms). Saturated fats increase blood cholesterol, unsaturated fatty acids seem to have no effect (there is some evidence that they may be beneficial), and polyunsaturates decrease cholesterol levels. However, too much polyunsaturate may create other problems not related to atherosclerosis; no one is sure.

Some vegetable oils contain large amounts of polyunsaturates. Others, like coconut oil and palm oil, are practically all saturated and almost as atherogenic as animal fat. Animal fat is mostly saturated. The words "partly hydrogenated" mean that some of the original unsaturated and polyunsaturated character has been destroyed by addition of hydrogen. This is done to make the final fat more nearly solid.

There is currently some interest in fish oil as a dietary supplement to decrease the risk of ischemic heart disease. It has been observed that some Greenland Eskimos have very low rates of this problem. These Eskimos eat a great deal of fish. Fish oils contain polyunsaturated fats with even more double bonds per molecule (5 and 6) than do vegetable oils. In addition, the double bonds are in different locations. Fish oils have a definite aspirin-like effect in decreasing platelet clumping (chapter VIII). In larger amounts they lower blood cholesterol. The advisability and safety of using these oils is still being investigated.

There are additional poorly understood effects of individual foods. A vegetarian diet appears to have a cholesterol-lowering effect apart from its fat content. Vegetarians have a higher HDL to LDL ratio than meat eaters; almost everyone agrees that this is beneficial as far as ischemic heart disease is concerned. Skim milk lowers cholesterol; low fat milk and yogurt, which contain some saturated fat and cholesterol, do not appear to raise blood cholesterol.

The National Institute of Health convened a panel of experts on this subject in November 1984. After evaluating all of the above factors and many more, they recommend that no more than 30% of our calories come from fat as opposed to the 40% or so in most of our diets now. They further recommend that no more than 1/3 of this be animal fat and that 1/3 but no more be polyunsaturates. Each gram of fat yields 9 calories; we get 4 calories from each gram of protein or carbohydrate. This recommendation then means a diet with no more than 1 gm of fat for every 5 or 6 grams of protein and carbohydrate combined. The NIH also recommends that total cholesterol intake be limited to 250 to 300 milligrams daily and that obesity be controlled by decreasing total calorie intake.

All this is likely to be quite a struggle in many cases. However, for the person with ischemic heart disease, control of diet and other risk factors presents a real opportunity—probably the only opportunity—to arrest or even reverse the progress of his illness. We must never lose sight of the fact that practically all of the treatment methods described in chapter VIII are exercises in closing the barn door after a large share of the livestock have been stolen. They are ways of trying to avert or treat a disaster; they do nothing about the fundamental problem, which is the progression of atherosclerosis itself. A good start for anyone interested is the American Heart Association Cookbook, which translates recommendations to recipes.

There are medications which lower blood cholesterol. They are very useful in patients with high levels (above the 260 range). All have side effects in some people. New ones which are more effective and apparently give fewer difficulties are now being used. No one can yet be sure about long range problems, if any. It would be desirable to have everyone's cholesterol at the level recommended by the NIH. However, even if there are no harmful properties, it might not be possible to get apparently healthy people with cholesterol levels near "normal" to take these medications for a lifetime.

G. Obesity

Obesity as a risk factor for ischemic heart disease has been the subject of a good deal of debate. Some studies show that people weighing up to 20% more than the maximum desirable amount shown on the usual weight charts do as well or better than thinner individuals. As an example, a 5 foot 8 inch medium-frame man could weigh as much as 190 pounds instead of the top weight of 157 pounds the charts now give. The question is not settled, except that nearly everyone agrees that anything over 20% above the usual figures is too much.

Some individuals tolerate obesity well. On the other hand, there are people who at some level of increased weight will develop diabetes, high blood pressure, and/or high blood cholesterol. Weight reduction will reduce or eliminate the problems in such people. Certainly, anyone with ischemic heart disease should keep his weight where his doctor asks him to.

H. Exercise

The question of exercise provokes even more argument than obesity. It has proved very hard to do controlled studies comparing exercisers and nonexercisers over long periods of time. There have been studies of large groups of free living individuals with different exercise levels. About half of the studies show a definite benefit from exercise and half do not. A number of problems make interpretation of the results difficult. In some cases other risk factors may overshadow any exercise effect. It is hard to tell how much exercise individual members of a large group are actually doing. There is the problem of self selection; are people fit because they exercise or do they exercise because they are fit?

It it well established that exercise increases HDL levels (section F, this chapter). It is also well established that elevated HDL levels are associated with less ischemic heart disease. This does not necessarily mean that exercising to increase HDL levels will result in less ischemic heart disease. There is always the possibility that there is an unknown factor sometimes but not always associated with elevated HDL and that it is this factor and not HDL that is responsible for the beneficial effect.

One animal experiment provides strong evidence that exercise does decrease coronary atherosclerosis. Monkeys eating their usual foods do not develop appreciable amounts of atherosclerosis. In the experiment 2 groups of monkeys were fed a special diet containing added cholesterol and saturated fat to increase their blood cholesterol levels. One group of monkeys was exercised on treadmills; the other group was not. After 24 months the exercise group had much less coronary atherosclerosis and much larger coronary arteries than the sedentary group.

It is most likely that exercise does decrease ischemic heart disease. Probably any exercise is better than no exercise. Measurable increases in HDL begin to show up after 9 months at energy expenditures of 500 to 800 calories per week; this is the equivalent of walking or jogging 6 to 10 miles per week. There are indications that benefits increase up to 2000 calories per week, but not much beyond that.

Exercise carries some risk. It is estimated that there is about one cardiac death for every 390,000 hours of jogging. In the great majority of instances there has been a preexisting heart problem that the jogger may or may not have been aware of. Much more common are sprains, strains, bruises, joint problems, and an occasional broken bone. Everyone should have a physical examination before starting an exercise program. Anyone with heart or other medical problems should exercise under strict medical supervision.

From there on the best advice is to do whatever exercise can be reasonably tolerated or hopefully even enjoyed. The hardest part of any program is the first few weeks. Most people, if they can get through the initial rough time, find that they feel better and function better if they exercise.

I. Personality and ischemic heart disease

There is some indication that there is a connection between the so-called type A personality and ischemic heart disease. The type A person is described as ambitious, competitive, and work oriented. He is obsessed with deadlines and always trying to accomplish more and more in less and less time. A study of 3,154 men over 8 years concluded that those with type A personality had twice as much ischemic heart disease as the more relaxed type B individuals. Other studies, however, have found no difference in type A and type B people.

There is a good deal of disagreement about the importance of these observations. Certainly, everyone should avoid as much unnecessary stress as possible. The desirability and practicality of trying to make extensive personality and behavior changes has not been established.

J. Conclusion

This discussion of risk factors probably represents majority opinions in most cases. On the other hand, there is almost no conclusion stated that will not be challenged by a number of sincere and knowledgeable individuals. In particular, some studies of people on cholesterol lowering diets have shown decreases in ischemic heart disease mortality but no change in overall mortality. The drop in ischemic heart disease mortality is balanced by other kinds of deaths, but not always the same kinds. In one study it was cancer; in another it was suicide. No one knows the significance of these findings, if any.

In this connection we should note that for the past 20 years the people of the U.S. appear to have been engaged in an experiment of their own. They have been exercising more, smoking less, eating more vegetables and less animal fat and cholesterol, and at least making some attempt to control high blood pressure. For this period there has been a 39% drop in death rate from ischemic heart disease and an even more striking drop in stroke mortality. Except for lung diseases, where the change is easily accounted for by past smoking habits, there has been no significant rise in death rate from any cause. It is evident that the health habit changes in the general population so far are safe. The death rate drop is saving around 400,000 lives a year.

As with any epidemiologic study, no one can "prove" a

cause and effect relationship. Improved medical care is responsible for some of the drop in death rate. The major part, however, is almost certainly the result of risk factor control. There is still argument about which risk factors are most important. It would seem that the prudent individual, whether he has ischemic heart disease or not, would do the best he reasonably can to control all of them.

GLOSSARY

Many of the words and expressions in the glossary have a number of meanings. The definitions and explanations here are for the way they are used in this book.

GLOSSARY

ACLS—abbreviation for advanced cardiac life support

AV node—abbreviation for atrioventricular node

abdomen—body cavity between chest and hips; contains stomach, intestine, liver, spleen, and other organs

acute—relatively sudden change in condition; depending on context sudden can mean anything from seconds to days but usually not weeks or longer

adrenergic agents—a group of chemicals having some of the same actions as some substances produced by the adrenal glands and some nerve endings; may have alpha adrenergic effects (mainly blood vessel constriction) and/or beta adrenergic effects, for which see beta adrenergic agents

advanced cardiac life support—American Heart Association protocols for restarting and maintaining effective heartbeat in cases of cardiac arrest and other severe rhythm disturbances; involves use of intravenous drugs, endotracheal intubation or other airway control measures, electrical shock as needed

alveoli (singular alveolus)—terminal small air sacs in the lungs (about 0.1 to 0.3 mm in diameter) where blood picks up oxygen from and loses carbon dioxide to air

anatomy—description of how the organs of the body are constructed, where they are located, and how they are connected

aneurysm—weak area in the wall of an artery or wall of the heart; may bulge or appear as blood burrowing between the layers of the arterial wall (dissecting aneurysm)

angina—short for angina pectoris

angina pectoris—chest pain due to inadequate blood supply to part of the heart, most commonly caused by coronary artery atherosclerosis; inadequate blood supply can be reversed without gross permanent cardiac damage, in contradistinction to myocardial infarction, where there is permanent damage

angiography—taking pictures of blood vessels, usually by injecting contrast media into the blood stream to allow vessels to be outlined on film by x-ray

angioplasty—procedure to change the size or shape of a blood vessel; usually done to increase blood carrying capacity

angioscopy—looking into the blood vessels of living people, currently by means of long flexible bundles of very thin glass rods

antidysrhythmic agents—drugs used to control or prevent abnormal heart rhythms (fast, slow, irregular, or arrest)

aorta—the single large blood vessel taking blood from the heart (left ventricle) and branching to supply the entire body

aortic balloon—plastic balloon placed into the aorta, connected to a gas supply, and synchronized to inflate and deflate with each heartbeat; helps the failing heart pump blood; for temporary emergency use (up to 2 weeks)

aortic valve—thin flaps of tissue at the junction of the left ventricle and aorta which keep aortic blood from running back into the heart when the ventricle relaxes

arbitrary—decision based on value judgment rather than facts or strong objective evidence; made because the nature of the problem precludes decision on facts, facts not available, or decider ignores facts; therefore subject to prejudice and whim

arrest—the cessation of coordinated ventricular beat and therefore the cessation of blood circulation; due to ventricular fibrillation or ventricular asystole

artery—any blood vessel or branch carrying blood away from the heart down to the very small ones, which are called arterioles; arterioles feed into capillaries

arteriography—angiography restricted to arteries

artifact—a change in a record or film due to operator error, machine malfunction, electrical interference, or similar problem and not due to biological change in the subject being tested

asystole—complete absence of contraction of any part of the ventricular muscle

atheroma—mass of crystals of cholesterol and related substances deposited in the wall of an artery together with tissue reaction to the deposit; the atherosclerotic plaque

atherosclerosis—disease characterized by the deposit of cholesterol and related substances in the inner walls of the arteries

atom—the smallest particle of a chemical element having the characteristics of that element; any further breakdown gives subatomic particles like electrons, which are common to all elements

atrial fibrillation—uncoordinated contractions of small bundles of atrial muscle resulting in "bag of worms" type of activity but no coordinated contraction; can occur in short episodes in normal people, frequently compatible with many years of active life even when present with heart disease; distinguish from ventricular fibrillation, which causes death in a few minutes if not reversed

atrioventricular node—specialized small nodule of tissue at junction of atrium and ventricles that is the beginning of the normal pathway for conduction of electrical impulses from atrium to ventricles

atrium (plural atria)—thin walled sacs of cardiac muscle that receive blood from the body (right atrium) and lungs (left atrium) for passage to the ventricles; 2 of the 4 chambers of the heart

balloon—refers to aortic balloon or balloon used for stretching arteries in percutaneous transluminal angioplasty (PTCA)

basic CPR—basic cardiopulmonary resuscitation

basic cardiopulmonary resuscitation—rhythmic chest compression and mouth-to-mouth breathing to oxygenate and pump blood in cardiac arrest; performed according to American Heart Association protocol

basic life support—basic cardiopulmonary resuscitation

beta adrenergic agents—substances manufactured by the body and by chemists, usually belonging to the chemical class called catecholamines; have a number of possible effects which may include increased heart rate, increased force of heart contraction, increased heart irritability, increased heart oxygen demand

beta adrenergic blocking agents—chemicals which counteract the effects of beta adrenergic agents; which effects and how much depends on the agent chosen

blind—in studies on drugs, single blind means the patient does not know whether he is getting active drug or inert lookalike; double blind means that neither the patient nor the doctor treating him knows

bronchioles—small air passages connecting bronchi to functioning lung tissue (alveoli)

bronchus—a major branch of the main windpipe (trachea)

bundle of His—bundle of fibers, specialized for electrical impulse conduction, starting at the AV node and going into the ventricles

bundle branches—the 3 main branches of the bundle of His

bypass—a blood vessel, natural or artificial, used to connect surgically 2 arteries to carry blood around an obstructed artery segment

cc—cubic centimeter; an inch is 2.54 centmeters; there are about 30 cc in a fluid ounce

calcium channel blockers—drugs which block the passage of calcium from blood into cells

capillaries—the smallest, thinnest walled blood vessels of the body; site where oxygen and nutrients diffuse from blood into cells and cell products diffuse in the other direction

calorie—unit of energy; energy (heat) required to raise the temperature of one cc of water from 15 degrees Centigrade to 16 degrees Centigrade (food calories are kilocalories, 1000 calories each); one gram of fat produces 9000 calories; one gram of sugar, starch, or protein produces 4000 calories

cardiac—pertaining to the heart

cardiac arrest—the cessation of heartbeat and pumping of blood; due to asystole or ventricular fibrillation

cardiac cycle—interval from the beginning of one heartbeat to the beginning of the next. Includes systole, then diastole, up to start of next systole

cardiac ischemia—inadequate blood supply to the heart

cardiac rhythm—rate, regularity, or type of irregularity of heartbeat

cardiopulmonary—pertaining to the heart and lungs

cardiopulmonary resuscitation—restoring the heart and lungs to function capable of sustaining life; see also basic cardiopulmonary resuscitation (CPR) and advanced cardiac life support (ACLS)

catalyst—something which speeds up the rate of a chemical reaction without itself being consumed in the reaction

catecholamines—a group of chemicals, amine derivatives of catechol, having adrenergic properties

catheter—a tube, usually flexible, used for injecting substances into or taking substances out of the body

cell—microscopic unit of body structure

central vein—superior or inferior vena cava or one of their main branches

cholesterol—a chemical compound of the steroid group, found in animal fat and manufactured by the human body; necessary for life, but it and related compounds can deposit in the walls of arteries to cause the disease called atherosclerosis

chordae tendineae—strands of connective tissue which anchor the free edges of the mitral and tricuspid valves to muscular projections from the inner walls of the ventricles

classical angina pectoris—one form of ischemic heart disease; characterized by pain with effort or stress, relieved by rest, and slow progression

clinical evidence—symptoms and signs described by and shown by the patient as opposed to tests such as x-rays, blood tests, and ECGs

cohort—a subgroup from a total population, the subgroup being those individuals under study or having the characteristic under discussion

collateral circulation—secondary blood vessels supplying a segment of tissue; assumes great importance when the primary supply is blocked

concave—curved surface bulging away from the observer

conduction—transmission of electric current or other impulse

congenital—present from birth

congestion—excess fluid present in tissue or organs

contrast medium (plural media)—substances which block x-rays to allow outlining of hollow structures on film

convex—curved surface bulging toward the observer

coronary—referring to the coronary arteries

coronary angioplasty—process using a balloon to widen the channels of coronary arteries that have been narrowed by atherosclerosis

coronary arteries—arteries supplying blood to the heart

coronary bypass—surgical operation to connect a blood vessel to the aorta on one side and the coronary artery system downstream from an obstruction on the other side; used to supply blood to part of the heart blocked off by the obstruction; the connecting vessel is usually a vein removed from the leg (saphenous vein) or an artery from the chest wall (internal mammary artery)

coronary heart disease—inadequate blood supply to the heart caused by narrowing of the coronary arteries, usually by atherosclerosis; practically the same as ischemic heart disease

coronary ostia—openings of the coronary arteries into the aorta

cubic centimeter—see cc

cusp—a valve leaflet

death rate—usually number of deaths per 100,000 people per year; may be given for specific ages, sexes, periods, etc.

diabetes—disease characterized by inability of body to burn sugar and other carbohydrates properly

diameter—largest straight line distance across a circle

diaphragm—thin layer of muscle and connective tissue separating chest from abdomen on each side

diastole—filling phase of cardiac cycle as heart muscle relaxes; happens once each cardiac cycle

diastolic pressure—blood pressure in the arteries during diastole

digital subtraction angiography—pictures of blood vessels made by taking x-rays of part of the body and computer-subtracting them from x-rays made with contrast media

dilating—increasing the inside diameter

dissecting aneurysm—blood coming through a crack in the inner wall of an artery (usually the aorta) and separating the layers of the arterial wall

double blind—see blind

dysrhythmia—any change from normal regular heart rhythm

ECG—abbreviation for electrocardiogram

echocardiogram—pictorial representation of parts of the heart built up by computer from reflections of sound waves; pictures are derived from series of boundary reflections and do not look like the heart

electric shock—a very carefully measured and administered amount of electrical energy delivered to the heart to attempt to convert arrest or a serious dysrhythmia to a normal rhythm

electrocardiograph—a machine for making electrocardiograms

electrocardiogram—a graphic tracing representing the changes in voltage produced by the heart during its action

embolus—a blood clot which has broken off, traveled in the blood stream, and lodged at a distant site

endarterectomy—surgical removal of the inner wall of an artery

endotracheal intubation—passage of a tube through the vocal cords into the trachea (windpipe) to allow controlled administration of oxygen to people with serious breathing difficulty

enzyme—catalyst which speeds up the rate of a chemical reaction in the body

esophagus—food tube which passes through the chest connecting the mouth to the stomach

evolution—development or passage from one stage to the next over a period of time

expiration—breathing out

fatty acid—chemical compounds which combine with glycerine to make fats; characterized by a long carbon-hydrogen chain with an organic acid group (COOH) at one end

femoral artery—main artery to the leg; its pulse can be felt at the groin

fibrillation—uncoordinated contraction of small muscle bundles of the atria or ventricles; heart chamber cannot contract normally when this dysrhythmia is present

graft—replacing (or replacement for) structure or tissue which has been lost or damaged; the substitute may be natural or artificial

gram—the weight of one cc of water at 4° Centigrade; there are about 28 grams in an ounce and 454 in a pound

HDL—abbreviation for high density lipoprotein

heart attack—frequently used for any kind of discomfort or symptoms in or near the chest whether they have anything to do with the heart or not; sometimes used to mean myocardial infarction; not a satisfactory term

heartbeat—usually the cardiac cycle starting with atrial then ventricular contraction going through the relaxation phase to the next contraction; sometimes the systolic (contraction) phase of the cycle only or the sounds produced during a cardiac cycle

heartburn—burning sensation in the chest, usually caused by stomach secretion flowing backwards into the esophagus; however, angina sometimes causes a burning sensation in the chest

hernia—defect in a body cavity wall, usually but not always the abdominal wall

herpes zoster—shingles; a virus infection, usually of skin and nerves only, caused by the chicken pox virus

hiatus hernia—defect in the diaphragm (upper wall of the abdominal cavity), usually the left, through which stomach or intestines can push into the chest

high density lipoprotein—transport particle for cholesterol in blood; apparently capable of removing cholesterol from plaques, so high levels in blood are desirable

His bundle—see bundle of His

history—everything the patient and the people with him can tell the doctor about his illness

Holter monitor—portable electrocardiograph that the patient wears during normal activity; can record electrocardiogram for 24 hours or longer to detect transient changes

imaging—making pictures or graphic representations

incidence—number of new cases per unit population per unit time, usually per 100,000 people per year

infarction—death of tissue due to inadequate blood supply; tissue is usually replaced by scar tissue

inferior vena cava—large vein which collects blood from the body below the chest and brings it to the heart

inflammation—swelling, tenderness, heat, redness of tissue, usually due to trauma (physical or chemical) or infection

inspiration—breathing in

internal mammary artery—artery of the chest wall near the breastbone (sternum) which can be used as a graft in coronary bypass procedures

intervention—any outside act intended to change body response or behavior

intestine—food tube in the abdomen starting at the stomach and ending at the anal opening

intraaortic balloon—see aortic balloon

intravenous—given into a vein through a needle or catheter

intubation—passing a tube into a body structure such as the stomach or windpipe (see endotracheal intubation)

irritability—capacity of a part of the heart for spontaneous initiation of an electrical impulse

irritable focus (plural foci)—segment of irritable tissue

ischemia—inadequate blood supply

ischemic heart disease—heart disease due to inadequate blood supply to part of that organ

LDL—abbreviation for low density lipoprotein

laser—very thin beam of light energy; can be used as very fine knife or to burn out tiny amounts of tissue, cholesterol, etc.

left heart, left side of heart—the left atrium and left ventricle

lipoprotein—an aggregation of protein, fat, and fat-like materials such as cholesterol; lipoproteins are the transport media for fatty materials which do not dissolve in water or blood

low density lipoprotein—the particular lipoprotein which transports most of the cholesterol in blood; when LDL is present in excess it deposits cholesterol in the walls of arteries

mgm—abbreviation for milligram

mm—abbreviation for millimeter

MI—abbreviation for myocardial infarction

micron—1/1000 of a millimeter; there are about 25,400 microns in an inch

milligram—1/1000 of a gram; there are about 28,000 milligrams in an ounce

millimeter—1/1000 of a meter; there are about 25.4 millimeters in an inch

mitral valve—the valve at the entrance of the left ventricle; this valve keeps blood from flowing back into the left atrium during systole

mitral valve prolapse—bulging of part of the mitral valve into the left atrium during systole

monitor—usually means a device used to show a continuous electrocardiographic tracing on a special TV (oscilloscope) screen or a recording instrument worn to tape-record heart electrical patterns over a period of time

myocardial infarction—death of heart tissue due to inadequate blood supply; dead tissue is usually replaced by scar eventually

myocardium—heart muscle; makes up the great majority of cardiac tissue

NMI—abbreviation for nuclear magnetic imaging

NMR—abbreviation for nuclear magnetic resonance

neurocirculatory asthenia—a poorly understood process and poorly defined term signifying chest pain, shortness of breath, fluttering in the chest with a mainly or exclusively emotional basis; not a heart disease

nifedipine—a calcium blocking agent useful in the treatment of angina pectoris and acute elevations in blood pressure

nitro compounds—drugs useful in the treatment of angina pectoris

nitroglycerin—the first and most widely used of the nitro compounds

nuclear magnetic imaging—imaging based on variations in spin and radio wave emission characteristics of atoms in a strong magnetic field

nuclear magnetic resonance—spin and energy production patterns of some atoms in a strong magnetic field; useful for imaging purposes as well as chemical analysis

nutrients—covers all substances, usually excluding oxygen and water, which an organism must take in to continue normal life and function

PTCA—abbreviation for percutaneous transluminal coronary angioplasty

pacemaker—either a segment of cardiac tissue initiating electrical impulses, normal or abnormal, to start cardiac muscle contraction, or an artificial device initiating electrical impulses for the same purpose

pain threshold—the level of intensity at which a stimulus begins to be perceived as pain; for example, the temperature at which something stops feeling just hot and starts to burn; varies from person to person

papillary muscles—cardiac muscle projections from the inner walls of the ventricles; connect to the free edges of valve leaflets through the chordae tendineae

parietal pleura—the inner lining of the chest wall

pectoris—pertaining to the chest

percutaneous transluminal coronary angioplasty—dilatation of narrowed coronary arteries by a balloon passed into the artery through the skin and aorta

pericarditis—inflammation of the pericardium

pericardium—fibrous sac surrounding the heart

peristalsis—a wave of muscle contraction passing down a tubular structure such as the esophagus or intestine; serves to propel the contents from one end to the other

physiology—the study of the function of body cells and organs

placebo—an inert substance disguised to look like an active medication

plaque—a collection of cholesterol, related substances, and fibrous tissue under the inner lining of an artery

plasmin—naturally occurring substance in the body which dissolves blood clots

plasminogen—substance circulating in the blood which, when activated by materials like streptokinase or tissue plasminogen activator (TPA), is converted to plasmin

pleura—inner lining of the chest wall (parietal pleura) or outer covering of the lung (visceral pleura)

pleurisy—inflammation of the pleura

pleuritic pain—chest pain characteristic of that caused by pleural inflammation; sharp, worse with breathing

pneumonia—infection of lung tissue

pneumothorax—collapse of a lung, partial or complete,

caused by air in the space between the chest wall and lung

polyunsaturated fatty acid—a fatty acid which has 2 or more double bonds in the molecule; helps lower blood cholesterol

predicted maximum heart rate—expected top heart rate (beats per minute) attainable by exercise; figures, decreasing with age, based on averages of maximum heart rates found in a large number of healthy people

prevalence—usually the total number of cases per 100,000 population present at a particular time; may be stated for a specfic sex, age, location, etc.

Prinzmetal's angina—angina pectoris due principally to coronary artery spasm

prolapsed mitral valve—see mitral valve prolapse

pulmonary—pertaining to the lung

pulmonary artery—main blood vessel taking blood from the right ventricle to the lungs

pulmonary embolus—a blood clot that has broken off from a distant site (usually the veins of the leg or groin), traveled in the blood stream, and lodged in the pulmonary artery or one of its branches

pulmonary infarct—a segment of lung tissue whose cells have died as a result of inadequate blood supply (usually due to a pulmonary embolus) and will be replaced by scar tissue

pulmonary valve—the valve at the beginning of the pulmonary artery as it leaves the right ventricle

pulmonary veins—vessels bringing blood from the lungs to the left atrium

pulse generator—the electronic instrument which initiates the electrical impulses for artificial pacemakers

Purkinje network—the network of fibers which, starting at the His bundle branches, carries the electrical impulses for cardiac contraction through both ventricles

radionuclide—radioactive element used for imaging

random—not according to any discernible plan or pattern; having no bias in a given set of properties

regression—shrinking, growing smaller, returning to an earlier stage

repolarization—the electrochemical recharging of the heart in preparation for the next beat

resuscitation—restoring activity or function

rhythm—the speed, regularity, or irregularity of the heartbeat

right heart, right side of the heart—the right atrium and right ventricle

SA node—abbreviation for sinoatrial node

saphenous vein—long vein in the leg frequently used as graft in coronary bypass surgery

saturated fatty acid—fatty acid with no carbon-carbon double bonds; presence in diet increases blood cholesterol

sensitivity—percent of all positive responders to a test who actually have the condition being tested for; "true positive" percent

shingles—virus disease of nerves and skin caused by the chicken pox virus; same as herpes zoster

signs—findings on physical examination indicative of a disease or disorder

sinoatrial node—a small clump of tissue in the right atrium which is the normal pacemaker for the heart

skeletal muscle—muscle attached to bone and used to move parts of the body; distinguish from smooth muscle present in arteries and intestine, and cardiac muscle present in the heart

sonocardiogram—see echocardiogram

spasm—abnormally prolonged and/or intense contraction of muscle

specificity—percent of all negative responders to a test who do not have the condition being tested for; "true negative" percent

stable—not subject to large and/or rapid changes

stable angina pectoris—angina pectoris which becomes worse slowly or not at all

stenosis—narrowing

sternum—breastbone; the bone that runs up and down the middle of the front of the chest

steroids—a group of chemical compounds characterized by a special arrangement of carbon atoms in 4 rings; cholesterol, sex hormones, cortisone-like hormones, and other body chemicals belonging to this class

streptokinase—a substance which activates a clot dissolving process in the body

stress test—a test in which a patient is subjected to gradually increasing loads of physical exertion while he is monitored physically and electrocardiographically to see if he shows any evidence of ischemic heart disease

sublingual—under the tongue, to be absorbed into the blood stream through the mouth lining

sudden cardiac arrest—cardiac arrest within one hour after the onset of a set of symptoms

superior vena cava—the large blood vessel which collects blood from the chest, arms, and head, and takes it to the right atrium

supraspinatus—the muscle across the top of the shoulder blade; it starts the motion of raising the arm to the side

symptoms—disease effects felt by the patient

systole—the contraction phase of the cardiac cycle

systolic pressure—blood pressure during systole

TPA—abbreviation for tissue plasminogen activator

tachycardia—rapid heart rate

tenderness—pain produced by externally applied pressure

tendon—bundle of connective tissue fibers connecting a muscle to a bone

tension pneumothorax—air in the chest outside the lung under enough pressure to move midline chest structures such as the large blood vessels to one side and interfere with blood return to the heart

thrombus—blood clot

tissue—any solid body substance

tissue plasminogen activator—substance formed inside the body, also prepared biosynthetically, which activates a body clot-dissolving mechanism

trachea—the main windpipe in the neck and upper chest starting at the Adam's apple and connecting to the lungs by way of the bronchi

treadmill—a motor driven belt platform used for patients to walk on in stress tests

tricuspid valve—the valve at the opening into the right ventricle which keeps blood from flowing back into the right atrium during systole

true negative—a negative test in a patient who does not have the condition being tested for

ultrasonography—imaging by the use of ultrasound

ultrasound—sound of higher pitch (air pressure variations of higher frequency) than can be heard by the human ear

unsaturated fatty acid—fatty acid having a carbon-carbon double bond in the molecule

unstable angina pectoris—angina which is rapidly getting worse

valves—flaps or leaflets of tissue inside the heart and blood vessels whose purpose is to keep blood from flowing in the wrong direction

variant angina—angina which does not follow the classic pattern of pain on exertion relieved by rest; sometimes used as a synonym for Prinzmetal's angina but may include other types

veins—blood vessels starting at tissue capillaries and joining to form fewer and larger branches; finally become the superior and inferior venae cavae emptying into the right atrium

ventricles—the 2 main pumping chambers of the heart

ventricular aneurysm—weak, bulging area in the wall of a ventricle

ventricular fibrillation—incoordinated contractions of small bundles of ventricular muscle giving the ventricles the appearance of a bag of worms; no blood is pumped, so this dysrhythmia is fatal in a few minutes if not stopped and replaced by coordinated heartbeats

ventricular tachycardia—rapid heartbeat with beats starting from an irritable spot in the ventricle; usually but not always serious dysrhythmia which may be preliminary to ventricular fibrillation

ventriculography—imaging procedures which show the ventricles

verapamil—a calcium blocking drug

visceral pleura—the covering of the lung

ORDER FORM

Colco Publishing
P.O. Box 35099
Houston, TX 77235-5099

Please send me _____ copies of Chest Pain—Is It Your Heart? I understand that if I am not satisfied I may return any book within 30 days for a full refund.

Name _____ Signature _____
        (Please Print)

Address _____

_____ Phone no. _____

Please enclose $9.95 per copy plus $1.00 shipping charge for the first book and 25¢ for each additional book.